pure scents for
Vitality

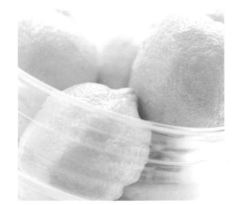

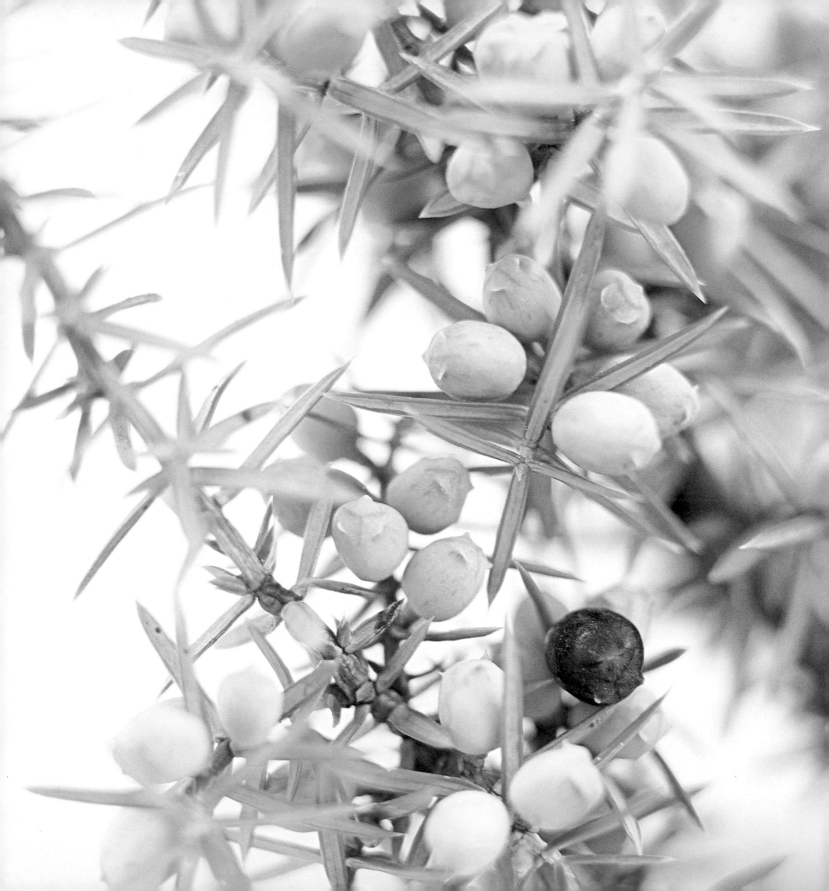

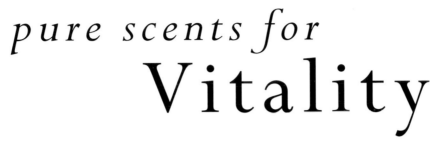

pure scents for
Vitality

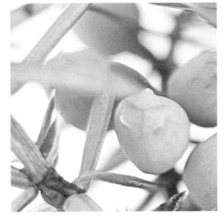

Joannah Metcalfe

photography by David Montgomery

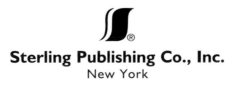

Sterling Publishing Co., Inc.
New York

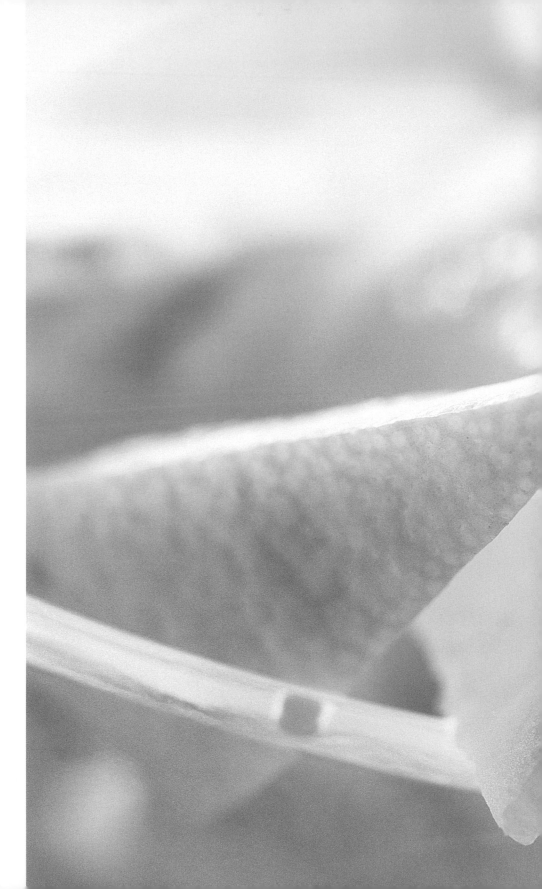

Publishing Director Anne Ryland
Designer Vicky Holmes
Editors Zia Mattocks, Jo Lethaby
Stylist Serena Hanbury
Location Researcher Kate Brunt
Production Patricia Harrington
Author photograph Henry Wilson

For my daughter Harriett

Library of Congress
Cataloging-in-Publication Data Available

10 9 8 7 6 5 4 3 2 1

Published in 1999 by Sterling Publishing
Company, Inc., 387 Park Avenue South,
New York, N.Y. 10016

First published in Great Britain in 1999 by
Ryland Peters & Small, Cavendish House,
51–55 Mortimer Street, London W1N 7TD

Distributed in Canada by Sterling Publishing
c/o Canadian Manda Group, One Atlantic Avenue,
Suite 105, Toronto, Ontario, Canada M6K 3E7

Produced by Sun Fung Offset Binding Co., Ltd
Printed in China

Sterling ISBN 0-8069-4815-9

**Before using any essential oils, please read
Aromatherapy practicalities (pp. 74–5) and the
contra-indications in the Directory of essences
(pp. 76–8). The application and quality of essential
oils is beyond the control of the author and the
publisher, who cannot be held responsible for
any problems arising from their use.**

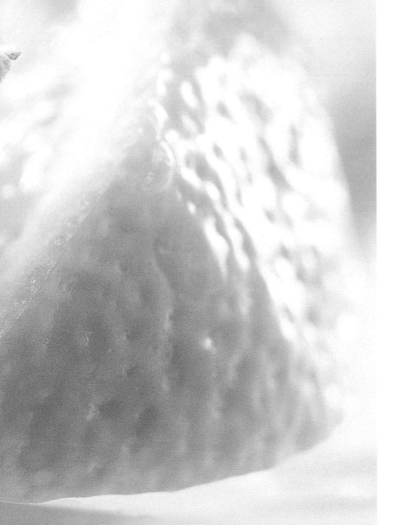

contents

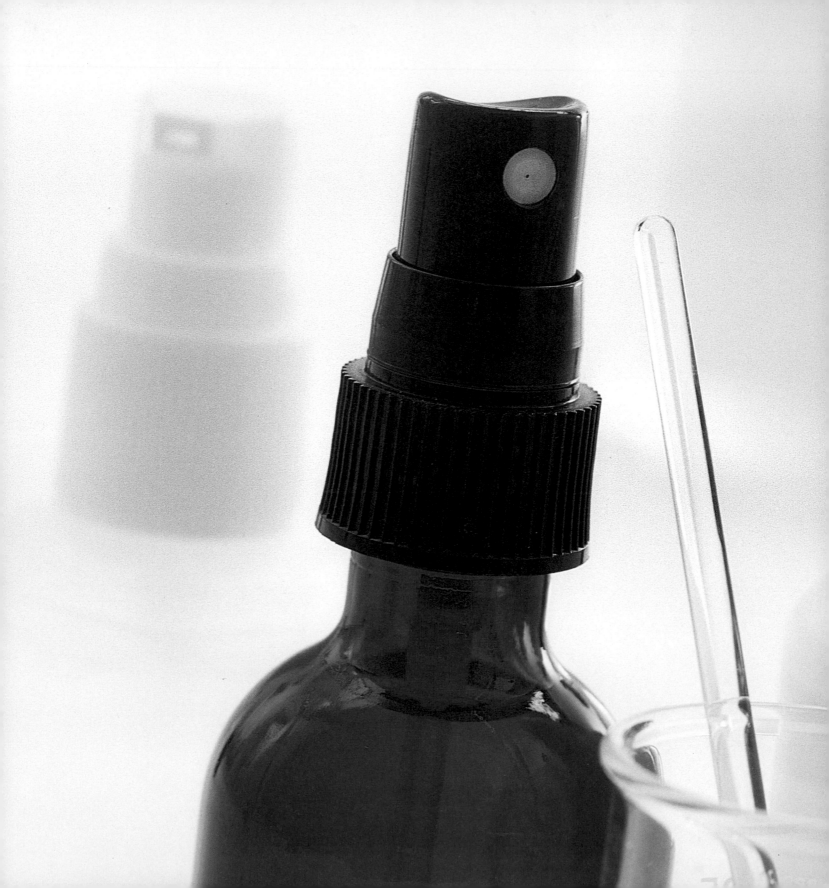

aromas for VITALITY

Natural essences can be used in endless

ways to stimulate our senses, reawaken

our bodies and minds, and create a

reviving atmosphere that will be both

physically and spiritually revitalizing.

Essential oils have been treasured for
their beautiful fragrances, medicinal
properties, and effects on the emotions
for thousands of years. Such uplifting,
relaxing, and stimulating properties were
probably first discovered by inhaling
the smoke from burning aromatic herbs
and resinous woods – the forerunner of
incense burning. Reflecting on the use
of essences through the ages gives us a
greater understanding of the enormous
wealth of knowledge we can draw upon
and apply with great effect to modern-
day aromatherapy practices.

Far Eastern cultures have an
uninterrupted tradition of using
nature's provisions for the restoration
and maintenance of health and vitality.
In China and India the oils were seen
to represent the essence or the force
of the plant and were used to enhance,
revitalize, or replenish lost energy, be
it physical, emotional, or spiritual. The
link between the mind, body, and spirit
was understood; and the plants, which
were highly esteemed, were used in
many different aspects of life, particularly to enhance and enliven mood and
emotional wellbeing. The Taoists,

aromatherapy past & present

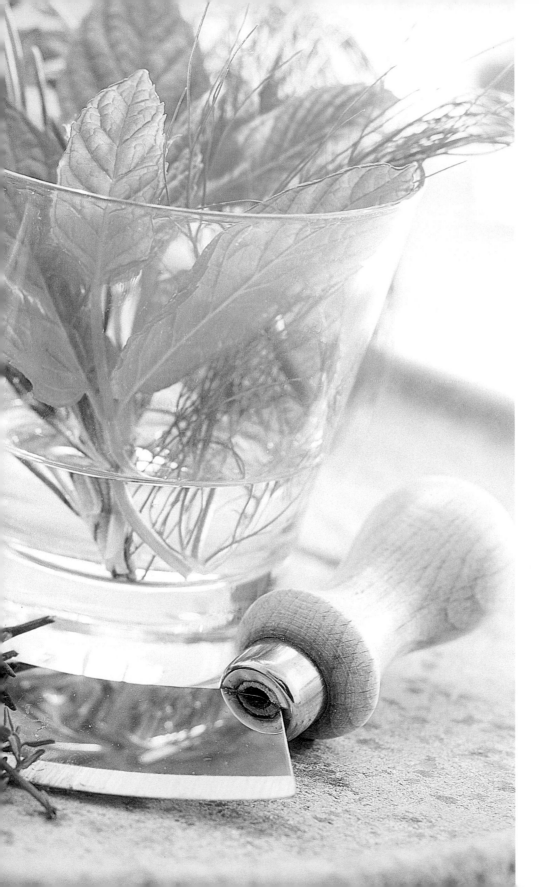

Hindus, and later the Japanese valued the use of incense in their temples and homes to engender whatever atmosphere, energetic effect, or therapeutic application they required.

Ancient Egypt is seen as the birthplace of aromatherapy. The Egyptians adored flowers, aromatic plants, and their essences, and used them in all aspects of life. Beautiful water gardens were created for the wealthy to retire to during the heat of the day. These gardens were a riot of color and fragrance, as aromatic plants from all corners of their empire were grown to delight and stimulate the senses. The essences were used as incense to scent homes and temples, and as offerings to the gods. Unguents, creams, massage oils, medicaments, and perfumes were part of everyday life. They scented their clothes, hair, and various parts of their bodies with essences that were often chosen according to the mood they imparted, as well as for their health-giving, deodorant or antiseptic effects, and to impart beauty, fertility, health, and vitality. The Egyptians set great store by the link between a happy spirit and emotional wellbeing, and used essences to transport the mind to other levels of consciousness. They also understood some aspects of the importance of diet and its energetic expression in the body, recommending fasting for some forms of poor health to give the body a chance to cleanse and regenerate itself. Incense and other aromatic inhalations, and the complicated formulas for medicinal and mood-altering combinations, were recorded on the walls of the stone chambers in which the high priests practiced their art.

The Greeks absorbed and developed the Egyptians' knowledge of aromatherapy. They used flowers in their natural

Essential oils have been highly regarded for thousands of years.

and distilled form, and draped garlands of flowers about the head and body to lift the spirits and exhilarate the emotions – rose and hyacinth were used specifically for their refreshing, revitalizing effects. Hippocrates, the "Father of Medicine," recommended daily aromatherapy massage and aromatic baths for long life, health, and vitality. The Greeks particularly prized unguents made from vegetable oils infused with aromatic herbs and flowers, such as thyme, sage, rose, and iris.

The Romans exhibited a more lavish use of aromatherapy than any other civilization. They used the essences in three different forms: ointments or unguents, scented oils, and perfumed powders. They particularly adored the cleansing, refreshing, uplifting combination of oils in bathing waters,

delighting especially in natural spa waters. They scented their hair and bodies, clothes, and bed linen; and they even applied fragrant preparations to the walls of their homes.

As Rome declined, the physicians and perfumers fled East, and the Arab world became the next center of knowledge for aromatics. The Crusaders then brought the exotic Eastern essences and the knowledge of how to distill them to Europe during the 11th and 12th centuries. This greatly increased the use of native herbs, and rosemary and thyme were joined by essences such as lemon, ginger, cedarwood, and sandalwood. The essences were much prized for use in perfumes to help relieve unpleasant odors at a time when even the most basic levels of hygiene were not used. They were also used to treat some maladies and to help prevent the spread of infection. Trade routes expanded, and the use of the more exotic oils and herbs swept Europe. Between the 14th and 17th centuries, many books – "herbals" – extolled the virtues of aromatic applications for physical and emotional problems, including the works of Nicholas Culpeper, which are still referred to today.

Paris had become the center of the perfume industry by the 19th century, and it was there that the link between scent and therapeutic effect was re-established. The term "aromatherapy" was introduced in 1928 by the French chemist René Gattefosse, who discovered the therapeutic effects of lavender essence when he burned his hand working in a perfumery. He plunged it into the nearest liquid, a vat of lavender oil, and was amazed how fast his hand healed, without scarring. This stimulated great excitement, and from then aromatherapy began to evolve into its modern-day form.

The beneficial uplifting, relaxing, or stimulating effect gained from inhaling the smoke produced by burning certain aromatic herbs and resinous woods has been recognized and practiced for centuries. It can help calm the nerves and emotions, ease physical tension, and aid meditation.

origins of
essential oils

An essential oil is a highly concentrated, chemically complex substance, which is derived from the flowers, leaves, wood, fruits, seeds, or roots of plants and is totally natural in origin. The essential oils, which are highly volatile, are produced by one of three methods – expression, distillation, or solvent extraction. Expression, where plant material such as fruit peel is simply squeezed, is the cheapest form of essential oil production. The majority of essences are produced by steam distillation, where the plant material is steamed at high pressure. The resultant water vapor is rich in essential oil molecules. Very fragile flowers, such as rose, are distilled by solvent extraction, an expensive and time-consuming process, because in normal conditions the heat would evaporate the delicate molecules. The macerated petals or flowers are soaked in solvents and then centrifuged to separate the essential oil from the wax and other waste materials. This mixture is then distilled gently in a vacuum at very low temperature to collect the pure fragile-flower essential oil molecules.

Ginger essence has a warming aphrodisiac effect, which promotes sensuality; lime is an uplifting and refreshing antidepressant; while lemon oil promotes a subtle spiritual awareness and eases mental conflict or confusion.

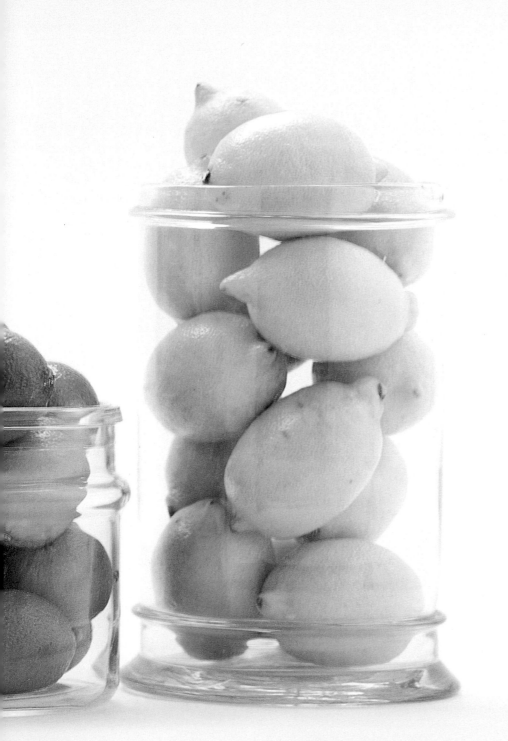

Essential oils have powerful, non-addictive, multidimensional properties, which can provide a valuable alternative to conventional drugs for relieving the buildup of stress, tension, anxiety, and depression, for example. They can help promote, maintain, and enhance our levels of energy and vitality in various ways. A congested, sluggish system is often reflected in low energy levels, and certain essences help to stimulate the circulation of blood and lymph, enhancing the body's ability to detoxify itself. They can also help stimulate the immune system, mental clarity, and concentration, and promote internal and external equilibrium (homeostasis). Essences can also be used on a subtle level to clear emotional and spiritual negativity, or to invigorate the atmosphere at home or in the work place.

The many ways scents affect us are as complex as the structure of essences themselves, and the study of olfaction has far to go before it is fully understood. This alone presents a strong argument for using natural products rather than their chemical counterparts, which can impart harmful side effects.

Essential oils enter the body by inhalation alone or by inhalation together with absorption through the skin. The majority should not be applied full-strength, but should first be diluted in water, cream, or oil. As the vapors are inhaled, the molecules are taken into the capillaries in the walls of the lungs and conveyed around the body as the blood circulates, where they act according to their individual properties. Many oils also have antiseptic and antimicrobial properties, which help relieve respiratory infections and congestion. The part of the brain that deals with memory and emotions is connected

inhaling & absorbing

directly to the lining of the nose by nerve receptors. As the essences are inhaled, this part of the brain is stimulated in positive mood-enhancing ways. Some essential oils stimulate and intoxicate the senses; others are calming and sedative.

For aromatherapy massage, essential oils are diluted in a blend of vegetable oils, such as sweet almond, olive, wheat-germ, or jojoba oil. The carrier, or base, oil reduces the concentration of essences; it prevents them from evaporating and allows them to be spread over a wide surface area. It is a moisturizing, nourishing, lubricating medium, which enhances the external layers of the skin but is not absorbed any deeper, whereas the tiny molecules of essential oil pass into the capillaries in the skin and from there into the bloodstream and lymphatic system. The essential oils are absorbed most quickly through the thin layers of skin on the scalp and face, and on the backs of the hands and feet.

Vegetable oils come from tiny glands in flower petals, leaves, roots, or seeds. The majority — and the cheapest — are highly refined, which reduces their odor, color, vitamin and mineral content, and therapeutic effect. The richer, more nutritive oils can be added to blends, usually in dilutions of 5–25 percent, to help certain skin conditions, including dry or mature skin. These oils are rich in antioxidants, which help prolong the life of blends by slowing down the oxidation process; adding oils rich in vitamin E also has this effect. The best-quality vegetable oils are the cold-pressed ones, such as wheatgerm or avocado, but a high content of crude vegetable matter can be indicative of high levels of fungal spores, which proliferate if added to water-based creams. Therefore, these nutritive oils are best used in massage-oil blends and stored in dark, airtight containers away from direct heat. Don't be

Some oils stimulate the senses; others are calming and sedative.

tempted to use synthetic man-made oils, as they will prevent the adequate absorption of essential oils, leaving skin sticky instead of silky, and they may also irritate sensitive skin.

Our energy levels can become depleted or compromised for a variety of different reasons, including our general life-style, diet, level of exercise, and genetically inherited predispositions. Essential oils and their various applications within aromatherapy can be used in a number of ways to naturally improve and maintain our energy levels and enhance our energetic potential, so that we function at our optimum levels of health and vitality.

Harmonizing essences, such as bergamot and geranium, help maintain balance and harmony, both in a literal sense within the body and also by imparting a feeling of emotional and spiritual accord. Certain essences, including juniper, lemon, fennel, and cypress help the body to detoxify and cleanse itself more efficiently. They assist and enhance the natural processes of renewal and repair, helping to free the restrictions or weaknesses resulting from congestion, poor circulation, and a sluggish lymphatic system. Many essential oils, such as rosemary, eucalyptus, lemon, tea tree, and black pepper, help the body by stimulating the immune system, which is often under pressure when our systems are stressed or overworked, and help fight infection more effectively. Some essences like peppermint and rosemary have a cephalic, or brain-stimulating, effect, which helps clear the mind and stimulate mental activity and clarity. This helps to relieve mental apathy or an inability to concentrate during periods of intense concentration or general fatigue. All essential oils help us feel as vital and energetic as we should by the very nature of their various healing properties, whether this is due to their general tonic effects or the specifically toning nature relating to specific organs, or to their cytophylactic (cell regenerative) actions. Examples of "tonic" essences, which help the body to help itself at many different levels, include black pepper, geranium, juniper, and grapefruit.

essentials on essences

Although the uses of essential oils are many and their therapeutic properties affect the body on all levels, before you invest in any, bear in mind that oils from fragile flowers are expensive, due to the process involved in producing them. However, these oils are so concentrated they need only be used one drop at a time, so they are sold in tiny affordable amounts. Most oils suggested for enhancing vitality fall into the lowest price range, and none are the very expensive fragile-flower essences, such as neroli, rose, and jasmine. Moderately expensive revitalizing oils are bergamot, black pepper, juniper, geranium, and ginger; the least costly are cedarwood, cypress,

Essences are affected by light, heat, and oxygen, and should be stored in a cool, dark place.

fennel, eucalyptus, lemon, niaouli, peppermint, pine, rosemary, tea tree, thyme, grapefruit, and lime.

Price reflects quality to a certain extent; and if you do find cheap oils, it is likely they will have been adulterated, either by chemicals, cheaper essences, or by vegetable oils. If you want 100 percent pure oils, check the label or accompanying literature. Some favorite terms for impure essences are "aromatherapy" oils or "natural" oils. Essences sold in clear or light-colored plastic or glass bottles are unlikely to be pure, since they react detrimentally to light and corrode most plastics. Organic oils are preferable, since they will not

have been tainted by any chemicals; they can be a little more expensive, although some in fact are actually cheaper.

Essences are affected by light, heat, and oxygen, so they need to be stored in a cool, dark place with their lids secure. Most oils keep for two years, depending on how often they are used: each time the lid is removed, the oil is exposed to oxygen. Oxidized oils look cloudy and should be used only for vaporization since the therapeutic action will be reduced. Citrus oils deteriorate at around six months (except bergamot, which can last up to two years) due to the high content of a terpene element, limonene, which combines with oxygen. Some oils, like sandalwood and rose, actually improve with age. Blends of essences diluted in a vegetable base that includes a little oil rich in antioxidants or vitamin E, such as wheatgerm or avocado, should last for two to three months if stored correctly, but it is better to mix small quantities at a time.

Use the essences individually until you are familiar with the effects of each, then make up blends using two to five oils; more than five detract from the aroma and effect. Perfumes are divided into top, middle, and base notes, and the ideal blend includes one from each group – although this is a guide, not a rule. Of the 18 essential oils for enhancing vitality (*see* pp. 76–8), top notes are bergamot, eucalyptus, peppermint, niaouli, lime, lemon, grapefruit, and fennel; middle notes are geranium, ginger, black pepper, juniper, pine, rosemary, tea tree, thyme, and cypress; base notes are cedarwood and cypress. Some essences can be categorized in more than one group, due to the different layers of scent that give them a multidimensional character.

mind, body, & spirit

Our levels of vitality and our general state of health are closely interlinked. While our lifestyle and diet are reflected very strongly in our energy levels, our attitude and sense of self also play an important role. Many of us feel constantly tired — mentally, emotionally, or physically — or feel spiritually drained and depleted. It is essential to take note of these various states of lowered vitality and remember that to resign ourselves to a life without a true sense of zest and vigor — a real feeling of *joie de vivre* — is to accept only half a life or less, as many of us these days tend to do.

Restoring harmony on subtle levels can enable our vitality to find its true expression.

Essential oils can be used to help alleviate stress, tension, and anxiety, which can all chip away at our defenses and deplete our energy levels. A constantly poor immune response is often linked to low energy levels, and the use of essences can improve and enhance our immune system, helping to prevent us from feeling low enough to succumb to infection and boosting our abilities to fight it off if it does occur.

The detoxification and cleansing aspect of essential oils, especially in combination with massage and aromatic baths, can initiate profound change on our physical, emotional, and spiritual levels. In aromatherapy massage, the oils that will help relieve poor circulation, sluggish lymphatic flow, or weak digestion are often indicated for the emotional or spiritual expression that often precipitates its physical manifestation. Many of us feel lethargic and listless for some time before we begin to become unwell, and it is at this point that action needs to be taken to alleviate the problem before it develops.

Many of the most revitalizing essences initiate a sense of harmony and promote many aspects of physical balance, thus restoring peace and encouraging the optimum operation of our internal repair and renewal mechanisms. The provision of ideal conditions to help the body help itself more effectively will often be directly reflected in an increased level of vitality and a general feeling of wellbeing.

When a demanding lifestyle and constantly heavy workload leave us feeling jaded and apathetic, essential oils can enliven naturally the aspects of ourselves that are most in need of refreshment. Stimulating essential oils, when inhaled or used in aromatic baths or in massage, can invigorate and reenergize us by stimulating brain activity. As mental clarity is restored and concentration is enhanced, the day can suddenly seem rather more positive than it once appeared.

Finally, remember that as we inhale and absorb essential oils into our bloodstream, it is not simply a chemical exchange that is taking place. We are receiving the pure vibrational essence – the life force of the plant itself. Restoring harmony on subtle levels can enable our vitality to find its true expression and help our lives to flow accordingly.

stimulating essences

Bergamot (not shown)
Citrus bergamia
The light green oil is fresh, sweet, and citrus with floral undertones, extracted from the rind of the fruit. Blends with cypress and ginger, and floral oils, especially geranium.
Antidepressant, antimicrobial, refreshing, harmonizing.

Geranium (not shown)
Pelargonium graveolens
A strong, sweet, slightly floral, pale green oil, extracted from the flowers and leaves. Blends with virtually all oils, especially bergamot, lime, black pepper, juniper, and rosemary.
Balancing, refreshing, diuretic.

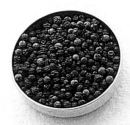

Black pepper (above)
Piper nigrum
A sharp, spicy oil derived from peppercorns. It is clear to pale yellow-green in color, becoming more yellow with age. Blends with citrus and floral oils, especially rosemary, bergamot, and geranium.
Stimulant, warming, aphrodisiac.

Cedarwood (right)
Juniperus virginiana
A soft, woody, camphoric, clear oil, extracted from the unused wood. Blends with bergamot, cypress, juniper, and rosemary.
Antiseptic, expectorant, relaxant.

Peppermint (right)
Mentha piperita
This very pale oil, with a strongly menthol, refreshing, minty scent, is derived from the whole plant. Blends with eucalyptus, lemon, geranium, rosemary, and tea tree.
Strongly stimulant, analgesic, anti-inflammatory, digestive tonic.

Thyme (below)
Thymus vulgaris
A warm, resinous, antiseptic, clean, very pale yellow oil, extracted from the leaves and flowering plant tops. Blends with lemon, rosemary, and eucalyptus.
Immunity boosting, antiseptic, circulatory stimulant, aphrodisiac.

Lime (below)
Citrus aurantiifolia
A fresh, citrus, green or pale yellow oil, extracted from the rind (expressed oil is superior to distilled oil). Blends with other citrus oils, floral oils, and rosemary.
Stimulant, tonic, antidepressant.

Lemon (below left)
Citrus limonum
A strong, fresh, sharp citrus oil, pale yellow to light green in color, extracted from the outer rind of the fruit. Blends with other citrus and floral oils, especially bergamot and juniper.
Antiseptic, immunity boosting, detoxifying, diuretic, astringent.

Juniper (left)
Juniperus communis
A clear to pale yellow-green oil with a clean, fresh, resinous, mildly spicy aroma. Top-quality oil is derived from the ripe berries; poorer quality oil comes from the needles, twigs, and wood. Blends with citrus and resinous oils, especially cypress, bergamot, and rosemary, and also geranium.
Detoxifying, diuretic, antiseptic.

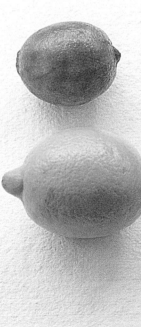

21

Tea tree (not shown)
Melaleuca alternifolia
A very pale yellow medicinal oil with resinous and menthol overtones, distilled from the leaves and twigs. Blends well with rosemary, lemon, juniper, eucalyptus, cedarwood, and pine. *Strongly antiviral, antiseptic, antibacterial, immunity boosting.*

Rosemary (right)
Rosmarinus officinalis
A strong, woody, menthol oil, clear to very pale yellow in color, distilled from the flowers and leaves. Blends with citrus and resinous essences, especially cedarwood and pine. *Strong stimulant, circulatory tonic, analgesic, aphrodisiac, antidepressant.*

Niaouli (left)
Melaleuca viridiflora
The clear, sweet, citrus, menthol oil is distilled from the leaves and twigs. Blends well with juniper, pine, cedarwood, thyme, and rosemary. *Stimulant, expectorant, strong analgesic, antiseptic, anti-inflammatory.*

Cypress (above)
Cupressus sempervirens
A pale yellow oil with a woody, nutty, spicy aroma, distilled from the leaves, twigs, and cones. Blends well with citrus oils, pine, and juniper. *Astringent, antispasmodic, decongestant, deodorant.*

Grapefruit (above)
Citrus paradisi
The refreshing, sweet citrus oil is pale yellow to light green in color and is derived from the rind of the fruit. Blends well with other citrus oils, juniper, geranium, and rosemary. *Detoxifying, diuretic, digestive tonic, astringent, antiseptic.*

Ginger (below)
Zingiber officinale

A warm, spicy, sharp oil, which is pale yellow-green but darkens to amber with age, extracted from the root. Blends well with citrus oils and many others, including cedarwood.

Warming, stimulating, aphrodisiac.

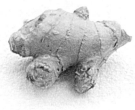

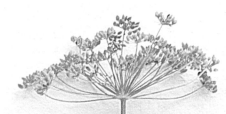

Fennel (above right)
Foeniculum vulgare

A clear to pale yellow oil with a warm, sweet, herbaceous scent reminiscent of aniseed. It is distilled from the seed of the plant. Blends especially well with geranium and lemon.

Digestive aid, diuretic, hormonal regulator, appetite suppressant.

Eucalyptus (above right)
Eucalyptus globulus

A colorless oil with a very penetrating menthol odor, distilled from the leaves and twigs. Blends with lemon, also woody, resinous oils like cypress, pine, cedarwood, and rosemary.

Strong stimulant, decongestant, expectorant, antiseptic, analgesic.

Pine (not shown)
Pinus sylvestris

A strong, fresh and resinous, clear to very pale yellow oil, extracted from pine needles, cones, and small twigs. Blends well with juniper, rosemary, and citrus oils, especially bergamot.

Stimulant, decongestant, tonic, antimicrobial.

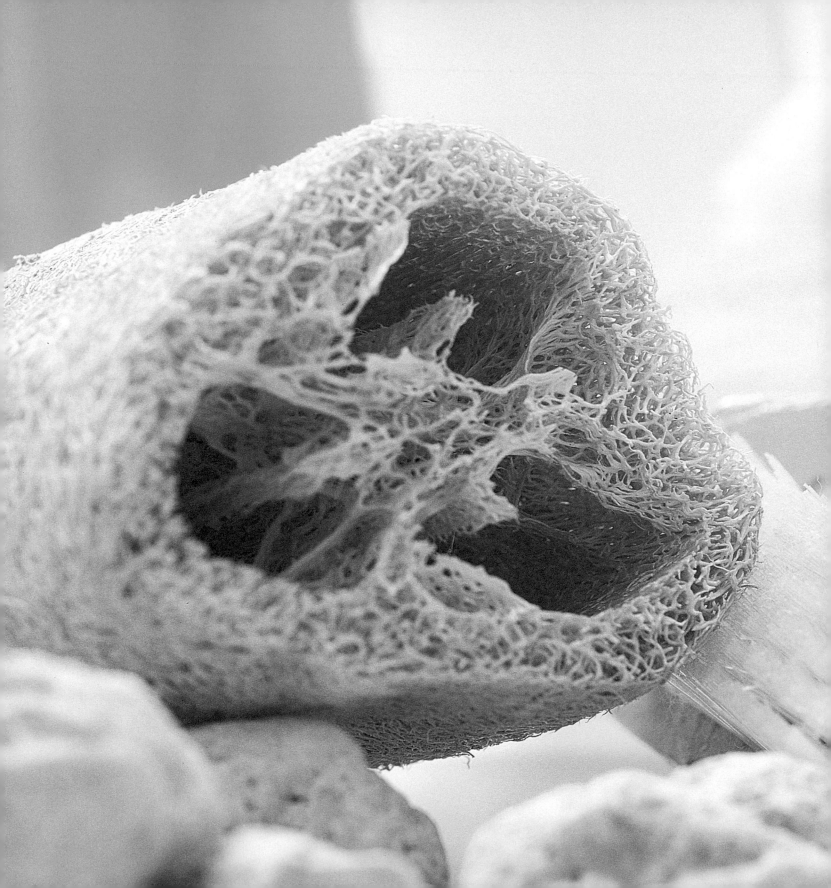

Invigorate the body and enliven the

mind by pampering yourself with

essential oils to help increase your

energy levels, maintain good health,

and enhance your sheer zest for life.

revitalize the
BODY

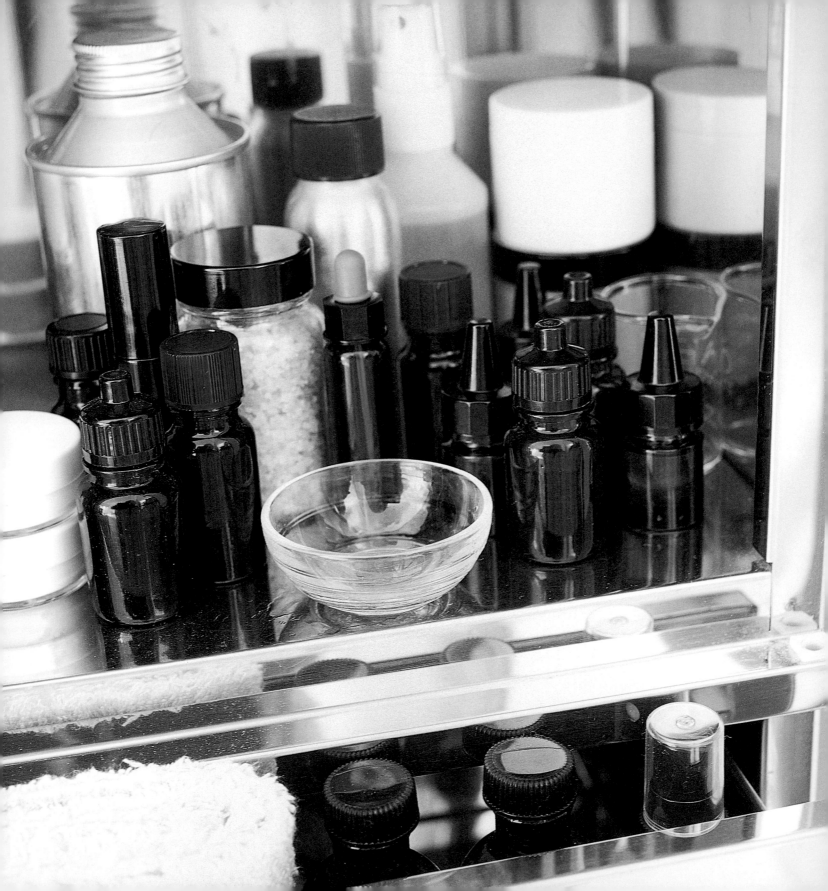

When we feel fatigued or uninspired by life, stimulating essential oils can help. Many of us mistakenly accept low energy levels, apathy, poor skin, tension, headaches, or low immunity as a part of life, but if we listen to these minor symptoms of "dis-ease," we are more likely to prevent serious ill health in the future. A little effort will help us attain the energy,

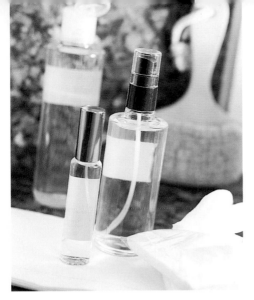

invigorate the body & increase

health, energy, & zest

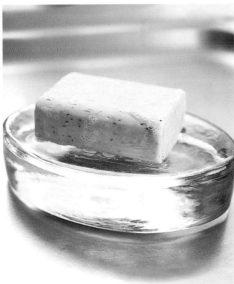

vigor, and zest for life that often seems beyond our grasp. There are some simple steps that can be incorporated into the busiest of lifestyles. With a holistic approach, everyone has the ability to slow down the aging process, feel fitter, younger, and more energetic; it is simply a matter of deciding that you are worth it.

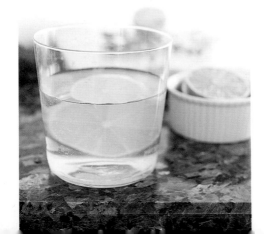

The body has the wonderful capability of giving us early warnings long before serious ill health manifests itself, and low energy levels are its way of telling us that all is not well and that certain aspects of our lifestyles need to be reconsidered. A little forethought and action now may save you a great deal of suffering in the future, and who knows what opportunities you may miss if you are too tired to make the most of life?

A certain amount of stress in our lives can be positive, stimulating our creativity, intellect, and ability to perform and achieve results, as long as we allow for subsequent calm periods in which to regenerate and recuperate. Stress becomes negative when it grows into a neverending cycle that is impossible to break. If we take care of ourselves, it is possible to counteract the effects and in fact to enjoy the stimulus

rather than sink under the weight of it all. Amid all the work and commitments that build up, you need to set aside a certain amount of time just for you. Depending on your pace of life and general state of health and vitality, you need time once a week or at least once a month for personal input, whether it is for exercise, creative pursuits, meditation, or simply to pamper and indulge yourself. This is essential for

relax & restore

keeping you happy and healthy and able to keep up with the pace of life.

There are various ways of helping alleviate the effects of stress and tension and thereby increasing vitality. Certainly, the essential oils used in aromatherapy can help refresh the atmosphere and the senses, and instantaneously stimulate energy levels. They can be used in many different ways, depending on the time you have and the degree of your fatigue. Aromatherapy is one of the most enjoyable, deeply relaxing ways in which to release emotional stress and physical tension. When you are deeply relaxed and your muscles have released their rigidity, your energy will not be wasted since your body will work with rather than against you. A relaxed emotional state also helps maintain a sense of perspective on life's ups and downs.

For those of us on our feet all day, a reflexology treatment is another blissful way of relaxing and revitalizing our systems. There are nerve endings and energy pathways throughout the body and in all major organs, which terminate in different reflex points in the feet. A reflexologist can stimulate the blood and nerve flow throughout the entire system, helping relieve the tension and congestion that can cause low energy levels, poor immunity, and subsequent health problems.

Traditional Chinese acupuncture, one of the most ancient forms of natural medicine, involves understanding the energy lines, or meridians, in the body and their relationship with our state of health. At an initial consultation seven pulses are felt and the quality of their energy assessed. Needles are then placed throughout the body to restore balance, release energetic blockages or weaknesses, and generally help the body function at its best. Acupuncture can be effective in the treatment of all sorts of "dis-ease" and may help those suffering from low energy and poor vitality.

A flotation tank is considered one of the ultimate forms of relaxation. It contains warm saline, which enables you to float in comfort, experiencing security and absolute relaxation. It can release tension physically, emotionally, and spiritually and restore a sense of peace and harmony relatively quickly.

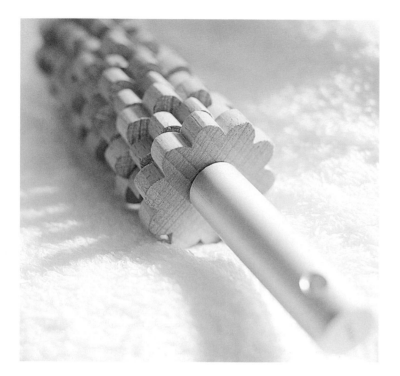

rejuvenating massage

Exercise, nutrition, and general lifestyle are all important for good health and vitality. Aromatherapy massage can also have a profoundly energizing effect, introducing essential oils into the bloodstream, so the essences can work their magic, helping your body feel its best and restoring your zest for life. The essences and massage techniques that speed up circulation and toxin release and stimulate the brain are specifically indicated, although a relaxant massage and combination of oils can also boost vitality by releasing stress, strain, and muscular tension,

thereby rebalancing compromised energy levels. Gentle, flowing massage techniques relax the system, while more vigorous actions have a stimulating, revitalizing effect. Your ability to breathe deeply and feel energetic again may be greatly enhanced by regular massage. Although a professional treatment may be advisable initially, the techniques and essential oils can be used effectively at home. It is most easily achieved with a partner, although you can massage yourself on areas such as the shoulders and the upper thighs and buttocks, where it is useful for helping prevent and relieve cellulite.

Begin a massage by soothing the back, neck, and shoulder muscles with gentle effleurage strokes, sliding the hands, palms down, up and down the area, following the contours of the body. Apply pressure only on the upward strokes, pushing the blood towards the heart. Next try easing deeper tension, to help re-educate posture and release energy blocks. With your hands facing each other as though about to clap, use a light but firm "chopping" motion downward so the sides of the little fingers come into repeated contact with fatty or muscular areas only, especially the buttocks, backs of arms, and upper shoulder muscles (trapezius muscles). Follow this "chopping" action with "cupping." This technique entails applying light pressure over the same areas, working with your hands facing down but slightly cupped as though holding a ball. The slight vacuum helps bring the blood to the surface and stimulates circulation. Always finish each of these sessions with more effleurage. Use the "chopping" and "cupping" techniques as a specific release for areas of congestion or tension — especially the upper shoulder muscles, buttocks, and upper thighs.

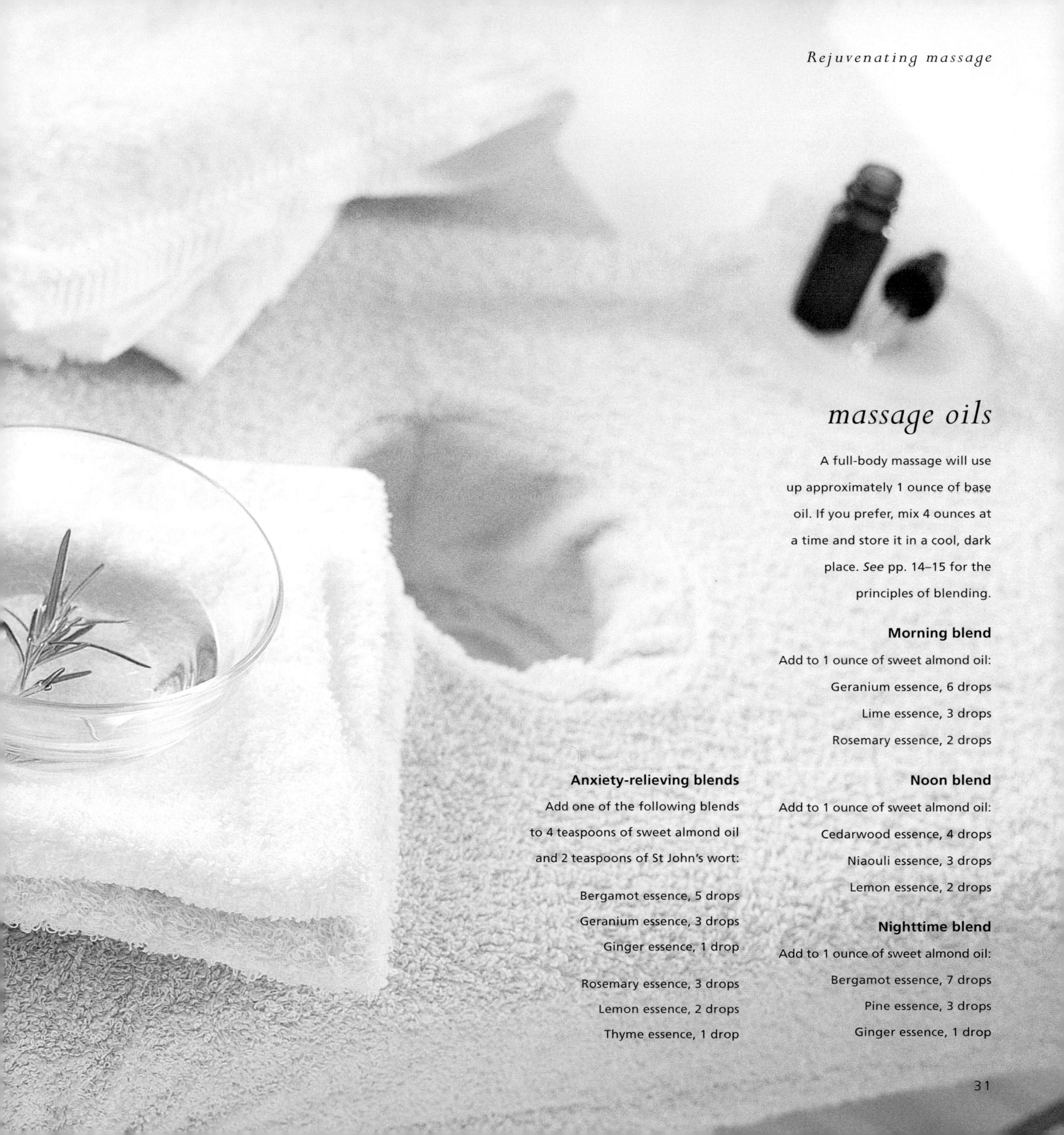

massage oils

A full-body massage will use up approximately 1 ounce of base oil. If you prefer, mix 4 ounces at a time and store it in a cool, dark place. *See* pp. 14–15 for the principles of blending.

Morning blend

Add to 1 ounce of sweet almond oil:

Geranium essence, 6 drops

Lime essence, 3 drops

Rosemary essence, 2 drops

Noon blend

Add to 1 ounce of sweet almond oil:

Cedarwood essence, 4 drops

Niaouli essence, 3 drops

Lemon essence, 2 drops

Nighttime blend

Add to 1 ounce of sweet almond oil:

Bergamot essence, 7 drops

Pine essence, 3 drops

Ginger essence, 1 drop

Anxiety-relieving blends

Add one of the following blends to 4 teaspoons of sweet almond oil and 2 teaspoons of St John's wort:

Bergamot essence, 5 drops

Geranium essence, 3 drops

Ginger essence, 1 drop

Rosemary essence, 3 drops

Lemon essence, 2 drops

Thyme essence, 1 drop

Although breathing is a natural mechanism that occurs without conscious thought, bad breathing habits negatively alter our levels of energy and vitality, our health, and even the rate at which we age. The entire body metabolism, circulation, nervous system, digestion and absorption of nutrients, and how we feel mentally and emotionally all depend on the correct balance of oxygen and carbon dioxide in the bloodstream.

As babies breathe in, they inflate the whole of the lungs, gaining the maximum amount of oxygen and releasing the correct amounts of carbon dioxide. Most adults breathe badly, and inflate only the top part of the lungs, moving the chest in and out rapidly to produce shallow breaths – especially in times of stress. Many health problems, besides constant tiredness and lethargy, can be linked to poor breathing, including headaches, palpitations, asthma, recurrent chest infections, anxiety, depression, and lowered immunity.

Learning to breathe properly can therefore be a big step toward improving your energy levels – zest for life is often enhanced as the body gets to work to its full potential. All the ancient civilizations had practices related to "power breathing." They inhaled herbal vapors and incense to encourage deep breathing and relaxation and enhance spiritual insight. Their exercises are used today in yoga, tai chi, meditation, visualization, and hypnotherapy. Both yoga and tai chi combine exercises and gentle stretching with deep breathing. Various self-help books can teach you the techniques (*see* p. 79). Practicing the exercises and inhaling essences can be the key to relearning the art of breathing. Once you have learned, try 5-minute sessions of deep, relaxed breathing to begin and end each day positively.

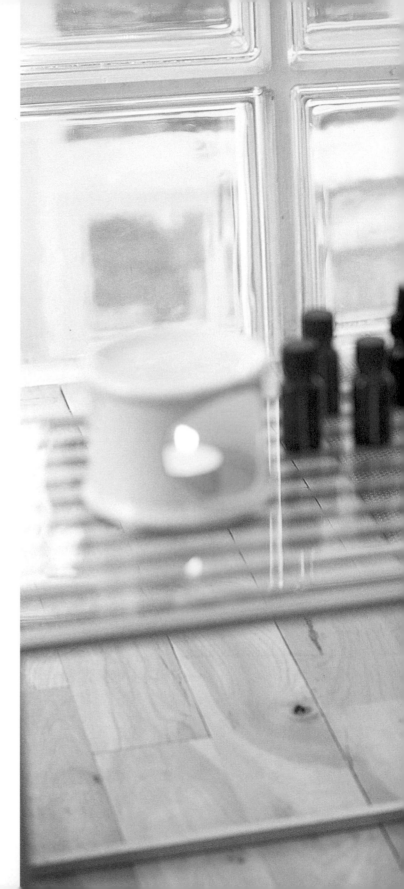

breathing for energy

Deep breathing

Vaporizing certain essential oils can assist the deep breathing process by helping you clear your head and focus on what you are doing, as well as boosting the immune system and cleansing the atmosphere around you (but do not use stimulants at nighttime).

Early morning refresher

To refresh and revitalize the senses and clear the head to increase concentration.
Grapefruit essence, 4 drops
Rosemary essence, 2 drops
Lime essence, 2 drops

Daytime uplifter

To lift the spirits, promote harmony and vitality, and cleanse the atmosphere.
Bergamot essence, 4 drops
Cedarwood essence, 2 drops
Juniper essence, 2 drops

Congestion reliever

A spicy, warming combination to relieve congestion and boost immunity and energy.
Rosemary essence, 2 drops
Black pepper essence, 1 drop
Ginger essence, 1 drop

Taking exercise is one of the most important ways of attaining or increasing vitality. It is one of life's ironies that you have to expend a certain amount of energy in order to acquire more. Exercise tones our muscles, including those in the heart and artery walls and the respiratory system. It stimulates the immune system and increases the body's ability to detoxify itself by improving circulation and lymphatic flow, stimulating

enliven body & mind

perspiration, speeding up digestion, and increasing the rate at which we release carbon dioxide and take in oxygen. Increased oxygen intake raises our energy levels. Exercise also elevates the mood and promotes relaxation and restful sleep.

A good way to relax and recharge is to engage in a sport. The exercise helps release any anger or frustration that has been suppressed during the day, and the activity absorbs your attention so you leave the worries and stresses of the day behind you. If you have fun exercising, the benefits are enhanced, and you will be more likely to keep doing it. Even a brisk hike can dramatically improve our health and restore energy and vitality, leaving us feeling recharged and revitalized on a very deep level. We breathe a better quality of air, and our senses are assailed by the peaceful sights, sounds, and scents of nature. Swimming, too, is an excellent form of exercise due to its gentle supportive nature and the fact that it uses virtually all the sets of muscles at once.

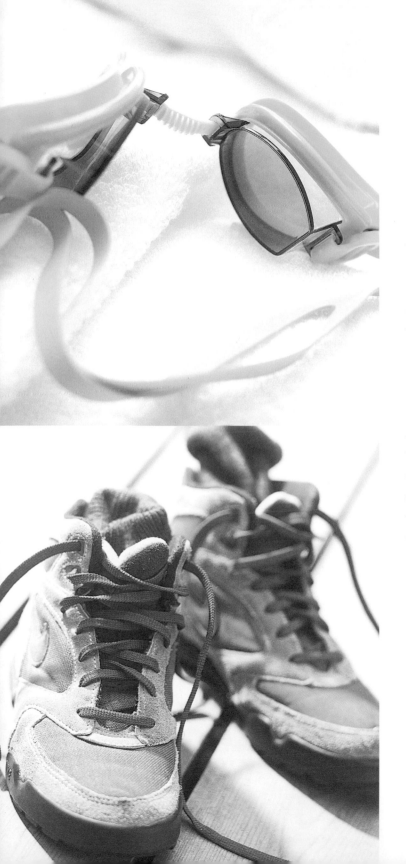

essential oils for exercise

Before-exercise massage oil

To warm the muscles and help prevent strain, add the following blend to 4 teaspoons of sweet almond oil and use it to massage the legs vigorously:

Pine essence, 4 drops

Rosemary essence, 3 drops

Black pepper essence, 1 drop

After-exercise massage oil

To help reduce any inflammation or muscle spasm and help prevent stiffness, add the following blend to 4 teaspoons sweet almond oil:

Cypress essence, 4 drops

Lemon essence, 2 drops

Rosemary essence, 2 drops

Eucalyptus essence, 1 drop

Muscle strain cold compress

For a strained muscle, add 1 drop of peppermint essence to a bowl of ice water and agitate. Place a piece of cheesecloth in the water, squeeze it out, and place it on the site of discomfort. Repeat regularly for 20 minutes. (Apply a few drops of undiluted lavender essence afterward to promote healing, ease pain, and lessen the bruising.)

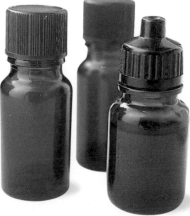

purify the body

*Drinking plenty of water
helps strengthen all of the
body's internal mechanisms.*

Water is essential for maintaining and increasing vitality, and it can slow down the signs of aging; it makes the complexion glow, the hair shine, and the eyes sparkle. It is needed to help our bodies cope with the demands put on our systems by the lifestyles we lead and the food we eat, yet most of us are always dehydrated. Water makes up a large part of our body, and every vital cellular function depends on the right balance of water and nutrients. Our brain is 75 percent water by volume, so our concentration, perspective, and mood can be drastically affected by dehydration. It also leads to sluggishness in everything from the minute cellular chemical exchanges to our overall vitality. When we are dehydrated, our body burns fat less effectively so we put on weight more easily. Congestion builds up so our circulatory system transports less oxygen and nutrients throughout the body, leaving us feeling tired and low. If we drink what our bodies need, we have higher energy levels, increased stamina and concentration, and less susceptibility to stress, anxiety, and exhaustion.

Our bodies lose on average the equivalent of eight glasses of water a day, so we should try to drink between three and seven pints daily. Drink one or two large glasses when you wake and plenty more throughout the day – not just when you feel thirsty. Interestingly, increasing your water intake does not necessarily mean you will be rising at all hours of the night; the body will have been more adequately detoxified during the day, so it will often have less need to rid itself of impurities during the night. Drinking more can also reduce water retention and puffiness.

Sadly, we live in an age where pure water is hard to come by. Tap water now usually contains a range of up to 2,000 different impurities. Carbon filters and reverse osmosis or distillation units can be effective in cleaning drinking water. Alternatively, bottled water can be rich in health-giving minerals, but read the label carefully as not all bottled waters are pure mineral waters; also mineral water in plastic bottles can be tainted by contact with the plastic.

Drinking plenty of fruit juice, tea, and coffee is most definitely not the same as drinking water. The point about drinking plenty of pure water is that it does not put any more strain on the body's filtration mechanisms, but helps strengthen all the internal mechanisms. Caffeine, on the contrary, is addictive and often causes headaches, sleeping problems, anxiety, and nervousness. It also raises blood pressure and stimulates the production of acid in the stomach. Tannic acid, found especially in tea, is another digestive irritant, and excessive consumption of tea can lead to an unhealthy intake of fluoride and a malabsorption of iron. Alcohol, in moderation, is enjoyable and relatively harmless, but taken too often or to excess, it drastically reduces energy levels, lowers immunity, and weakens our systems, especially the liver.

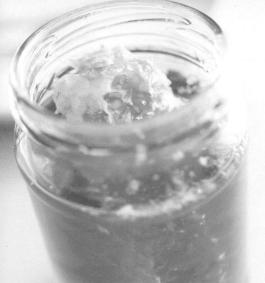

eating for energy

Natural herb teas are health giving and energy boosting, and drinking them is a safe way of ingesting and benefiting from the herb's essential oil. Peppermint and fennel teas are both digestive aids and natural diuretics, while ginger aids digestion and stimulates energy levels.

Early morning ginger tea

To make ginger tea add ¼ teaspoon ground ginger or finely sliced or crushed fresh root to hot water. Steep for 5 minutes before drinking.

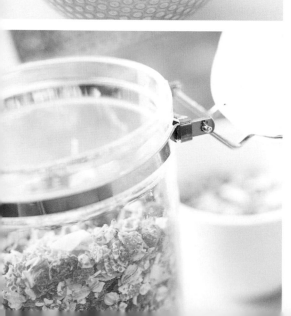

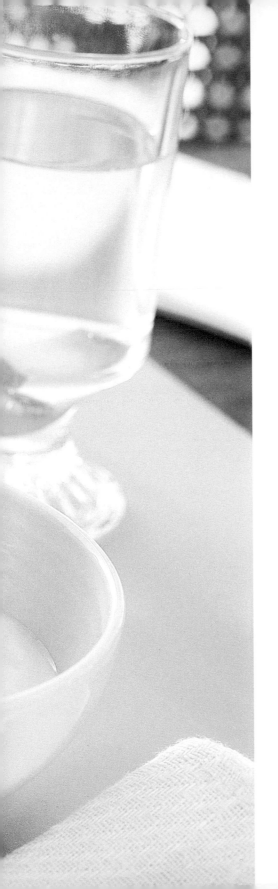

A poor diet leaves us low in energy and vitality, with our internal systems sluggish and congested with the toxins – chemicals, synthetic sweeteners, flavorings, preservatives, and excess salt – increasingly prevalent in our food.

The healthier alternatives include organic foods – free from artificial chemicals, they tend to be fresher and richer in nutrients, and help provide all the goodness we need. Replace white sugar with honey or brown sugar, and salt with soy sauce, miso, seaweed extracts, or a potassium-based low-salt alternative. Substitute good-quality cold-pressed olive oil for saturated oils, and replace margarine with an unhydrogenated alternative or a small amount of unsalted organic butter.

A balanced, healthy, revitalizing diet should consist of about 20 percent protein, 30–40 percent vegetables, 30 percent whole grains (brown rice, wheat, barley, maize, oats), 10–20 percent fruit and nuts. Try to stick to a diet high in fiber and essential fatty acids (found in virgin olive oil and oily fish) and low in sugar, salt, and saturated fats (cheese, cream, milk, red meat, and fried foods). To help your digestion, eat food slowly and chew thoroughly before swallowing, and do not drink too much with your meal. This forces the food down too rapidly, causing indigestion, and dilutes the digestive juices, making them less effective.

An intolerance to certain foods is increasingly common and may affect health and vitality. Classic food allergies include gluten (wheat), dairy produce (cow's milk, cheese, cream, yogurt), and yeast (bread, wine, beer). The Hay Diet, or food combining, can help solve some people's health problems. The premise is that eating "foods that fight" drastically reduces energy levels since they cannot be efficiently digested together and the process of breaking down and assimilating the food requires more energy than would otherwise be the case, and can cause other health problems and digestive weaknesses.

A short period of fasting can be a highly effective method of cleansing and reenergizing your system, gently increasing your levels of energy and vitality. It should ideally be carried out under professional guidance.

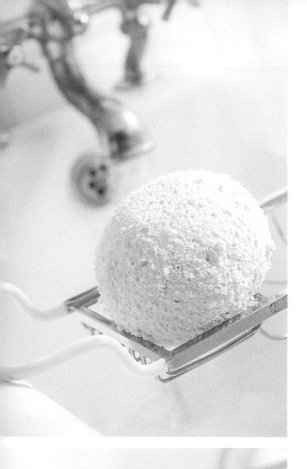

Aromatic baths are an effective way of using essential oils in the home, and pampering yourself is a revitalizing aspect of the experience. Add blends of essences (*see* opposite) to a teaspoon of vegetable oil or milk before adding to a full bath, to help disperse them fully. Relax for at least 20 minutes to allow the oils to be absorbed into your bloodstream and breathe deeply to inhale the vapors. To enhance the effect, vaporize the essences, or burn a candle until a pool of wax has formed, then blow it out and add drops of essential oil to the melted wax before relighting the candle. (Since the oil is flammable, take care not to drip any on the wick.)

For showering, add the same blends of essences, with the number of drops doubled, to 4 ounces of a natural, bland shower gel base. A particularly vitalizing aspect of showering is that you can alternate the water temperature between hot and cold, which stimulates the circulatory system and lymphatic flow, helping to tone and energize.

Skin brushing is highly stimulating and an effective way of increasing the body's ability to detoxify itself. It also enhances lymphatic flow and helps the body eliminate wastes through the skin. For an energy buzz first thing in the morning, use a long-handled, natural-bristle brush and sweep it over the body before you bathe. Use firm, regular strokes on the soles of the feet, up the legs, buttocks, back, and across the shoulders; from the hands up the inner and outer arms. Use gentler strokes across the front of the body and clockwise rotation on the abdomen to stimulate your digestion.

Hair reflects our internal state and lank hair can indicate low vitality. Add 4 drops of rosemary essence to two pints of warm water for a final rinse after shampooing to increase shine. A hair tonic twice a week is also effective.

cleansing & revitalizing

baths & showers

Morning

Use one of the following blends to refresh, reawaken, and revitalize the system.

Geranium essence, 4 drops

Lime essence, 2 drops

Rosemary essence, 2 drops

Bergamot essence, 5 drops

Cypress essence, 3 drops

Pine essence, 2 drops

Noon

For a midday boost that will restore, renew, and reenergize the body, mind, and spirit.

Cedarwood essence, 3 drops

Lemon essence, 2 drops

Niaouli essence, 2 drops

Night

To relax, release tension and aid recuperation.

Bergamot essence, 5 drops

Pine essence, 2 drops

Ginger essence, 1 drop

hair

Tonic for lackluster hair

A tonic twice a week will improve the condition of the scalp and hair and leave it smelling wonderful.

8 ounces orange-flower or rose water

1 tablespoon apple cider vinegar

Geranium essence, 4 drops

Rosemary essence, 4 drops

Juniper essence, 3 drops

Mix the ingredients in a glass bottle and shake well before use. Massage the tonic into the scalp and throughout the hair for 5 minutes, then shampoo as normal.

facial skincare

Honey & lemon facial scrub

1 teaspoon salt

1 rounded cup oatmeal

3 teaspoons milk

2 teaspoons lemon juice

3 teaspoons liquid honey

Lemon essence, 2 drops

Eucalyptus essence, 1 drop

Combine the ingredients, adding more oatmeal if necessary, to give a consistency thick enough to stay on the face without sliding off.

Blemished skin face mask

½ cucumber (with skin on), mashed or pulped in a food processor

1 teaspoon lemon juice

3 heaped teaspoons oatmeal

Tea tree essence, 2 drops

Geranium essence, 2 drops

Combine the cucumber with the lemon juice and oatmeal. Add the essential oils, then apply the mask to the face, avoiding the eyes. (Place a slice of cucumber on each eyelid for a cooling, anti-inflammatory effect, if you like.) Leave the mask on for 5–10 minutes. One drop of undiluted tea tree essence applied with a cotton swab can be used on spots after the mask has been removed.

radiant skin

Apple & geranium facial scrub

1 heaped tablespoon oatmeal

2 teaspoons mashed or puréed raw apple

Geranium essence, 2 drops

Juniper essence, 1 drop

A little water or apple juice to bind if necessary

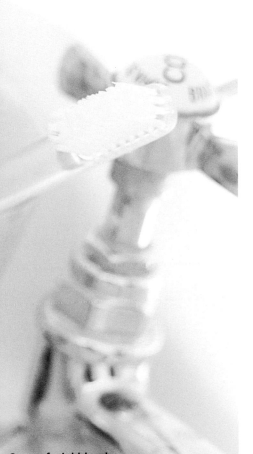

Skin lacking vitality and a healthy glow benefits from treatment that stimulates blood flow to the face and helps enhance the renewal and repair mechanisms that improve skin condition. Always cleanse the face of all traces of make-up first.

A face mask or a steam facial twice weekly will remove deep-down impurities and revitalize the complexion, but avoid steam facials if you suffer from thread veins or asthma. For a steam facial, pour hot, not boiling, water into a bowl containing your blend of oils. Lean over the bowl and place a towel over your head to trap the essential oil-laden steam. Close your eyes and stay there for 5–10 minutes, then splash your face with very cold water to help close the pores and stimulate the circulation.

Exfoliation two or three times a week (less for dry skin types) stimulates the removal of dead skin cells. Using gentle circular motions, apply a facial scrub, avoiding the eyes and concentrating on the oily areas around the forehead, nose, and chin. Leave for a few minutes, then rinse off with warm water. Splash your face with very cold water and pat dry with a towel.

Steam facial blend
Add to a bowl of hot (not boiling) water one of the following blends:
Geranium essence, 4 drops
Cypress essence, 3 drops
Lemon essence, 1 drop

A handful of fresh
rosemary, fennel, and thyme or
the essences (rosemary 3 drops,
fennel 3 drops, thyme 1 drop)

A handful of fresh peppermint leaves
or 1 drop of peppermint essence

Pamper yourself with a little "essential" attention

and give your skin a radiant healthy glow.

Refreshing skin tonic

Will help cleanse, refresh,

tone, and balance skin.

4 teaspoons witch hazel

1 ounce rose water

Geranium essence, 6 drops

Rosemary essence, 3 drops

Tea tree essence, 3 drops

Add the ingredients to a dark

glass bottle. Shake before use.

Apply using a cotton pad.

replenishing moisture

If you have taken the first steps toward revitalizing your complexion, such as a face mask, steam facial, or exfoliation (*see* pp. 42–3), your skin will benefit from a simple toning and moisturizing routine. Moisturizers are particularly beneficial since they help protect the skin from moisture loss and dehydration, assisting the maintenance of smooth, supple skin.

Wipe the oily areas of the face – the chin, forehead, and nose – with a gently astringent toner to help close the pores after cleansing and to prevent spots. Then moisturize with a light moisturizer before applying any make-up. During the day use a light liquid moisturizer containing essential oils to help enhance skin condition, stimulating skin cell renewal and repair. At bedtime, use a richer night cream containing vitamins and essences to enhance skin condition and repair the skin after the heavy demands of the day and to help delay the aging process. Do make it a part of your daily routine to remove all make-up fully before going to bed, in order to help keep your complexion clear and healthy.

Moisturizing balm

This can be used 2–3 times a week instead of your normal moisturizing cream, or in addition if you prefer to use one with sun protection factors.

1 teaspoon jojoba oil

1 teaspoon avocado oil

4 teaspoons sweet almond oil

Bergamot essence, 10 drops

Geranium essence, 5 drops

Combine the ingredients and shake well before use. Apply a thin film to the face, massaging it in with your finger tips. Leave for 10 minutes, then blot off the excess with tissues.

Light daytime moisturizer

5 tablespoons glycerin

3 tablespoons rose water

1,000 iu vitamin E tablet, crushed

Bergamot essence, 30 drops

Geranium essence, 20 drops

Add the ingredients to a dark glass bottle, shake well before use.

treats for
tired eyes

eye compresses

Essential oils should always be used with care on or near the eyes. They can, however, be used for refreshing tired or puffy eyes in the form of compresses applied to closed eyes for a few minutes while you lie flat or in the bath.

Teabag treatment

Make camomile tea with 2 teabags and infuse for 2 minutes. Remove the teabags, squeeze gently, and cool them. Squeeze out any excess water. Lie down and close your eyes, placing a teabag on each eyelid. Leave for 5–10 minutes. Remove the teabags and splash your face with cold water.

Tired eyes compress

Soak a square of gauze in a bowl containing 2 pints of cold water and 1 drop of camomile essence in 1 teaspoon of milk. Squeeze out gently and apply to closed eyelids and forehead.

Puffy eyes compress

Soak two cotton pads or small squares of gauze in rose water and place in the fridge. Squeeze out and apply to closed eyelids for 10 minutes.

foot baths

Before bed

For a warming, uplifting, soothing effect, add to warm (not hot) water, which covers the feet and reaches a level at least above the ankle bones: 5 drops of bergamot and 2 drops of ginger essence in 1 teaspoon of vegetable oil or milk. (Lavender may be added for painful feet or sleeping problems.)

Before going out

Fill one bowl with warm water and another with cold, to the level described above. To both bowls add the following: 3 drops of geranium, 2 drops of rosemary, and 1 drop of black pepper essence in 1 teaspoon of vegetable oil or milk *Soak your feet for 5 minutes in one bowl, then 5 minutes in the other, and repeat 2–3 times.*

For puffy ankles or feet

This may help circulation and release congestion (but is not for use before bedtime). It may also help arthritic conditions or gout, used in a massage oil. Add to 1 teaspoon of vegetable oil or milk: 2 drops each of lemon and cypress and 1 drop of eucalyptus essence.

Foot massage oil

A soothing oil to ease aching feet and stimulate blood flow. Add to 2 teaspoons of sweet almond and 1 teaspoon of avocado or wheatgerm oil:

Juniper essence, 4 drops

Rosemary essence, 3 drops

Peppermint essence, 1 drop

For tired feet that have been used and abused all day long, there is nothing quite so delicious as a foot bath. You might not have time for a bath or shower, but you can easily enjoy a foot bath while you are eating or sitting down relaxing, before you go out or before you go to bed. You may even like to try one of the small commercial foot spas available, which agitate the water and add to the pleasure.

put a spring in your step

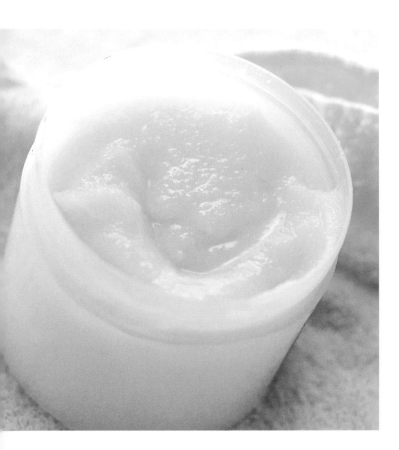

If your feet are tired, hot, and in need of refreshing, a peppermint foot spray is a wonderful treat. Add to an atomizer or plant spray 1 tablespoon of eau de Cologne, 1 tablespoon of rose water, and the following essences: 6 drops of tea tree, 4 drops of lime, and 2 drops of peppermint. Shake well and spray on your bare feet. Pat dry with a towel or let dry naturally.

If you have been on your feet all day and have swollen ankles or feet, they may need some attention if you need to carry on or want to go out. First lie on your back with your feet raised above the level of your head for at least 10 minutes. This aids venous circulation and lymphatic flow. Place your feet in a cold foot bath with 1 drop of peppermint essence. Leave for 10 minutes, then place your feet on a towel. Massage them with a soothing blend of oils (*see* above left) to ease the aches, help relieve water retention, and stimulate the blood flow. Last, drink at least three large glasses of water, since water retention can be partly due to dehydration.

For those especially low moments – the "morning after the night before" state or simply waking up exhausted and looking in the mirror in horror, try some revitalizing tips.

Drinking peppermint or fennel tea first thing in the morning with thin slices of gingerroot will calm the stomach and refresh the mind and body. Vaporizing 3 drops of rosemary, 2 drops of lemon, and 1 drop of peppermint essence will help clear the head and stimulate brain pattern and energy levels.

from overindulgence to exuberance

Revitalizing essences in the form of an aromatic bath or inhalation before breakfast will also help. Juniper and fennel both have a diuretic, detoxifying effect and will help your body eliminate problematic toxins more efficiently. Rosemary stimulates the circulation and energy levels and will help clear the head. Grapefruit is a liver tonic and has an uplifting aroma, while geranium balances emotional extremes and refreshes the senses. In addition, drink plenty of water, take 500–1000 mg of vitamin C, and eat little and often if possible.

To avoid those "morning after" feelings altogether, try drinking organic wine, which is less likely to result in a hangover due to the lack of chemicals. Alternatively, drink one glass of spring water for every glass of alcohol and you will not suffer such catastrophic consequences the next day.

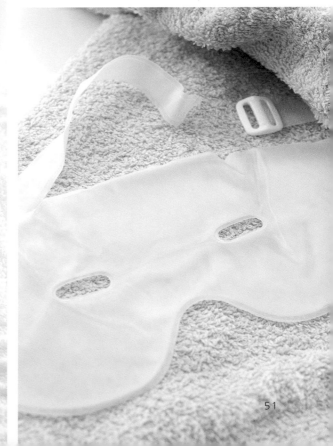

hangover cures

Have an aromatic bath or inhalation before breakfast – if you can face it – using one of the following blends.

Quick start reviver

For those who need to wake up, get "with it," and go to work. To 1 teaspoon of vegetable oil add:

Rosemary essence, 4 drops

Juniper essence, 3 drops

Fennel essence, 2 drops

Slow start reviver

For those who can take it easy and "come to" more slowly. To 1 teaspoon of vegetable oil add:

Grapefruit essence, 5 drops

Geranium essence, 3 drops

Fennel essence, 3 drops

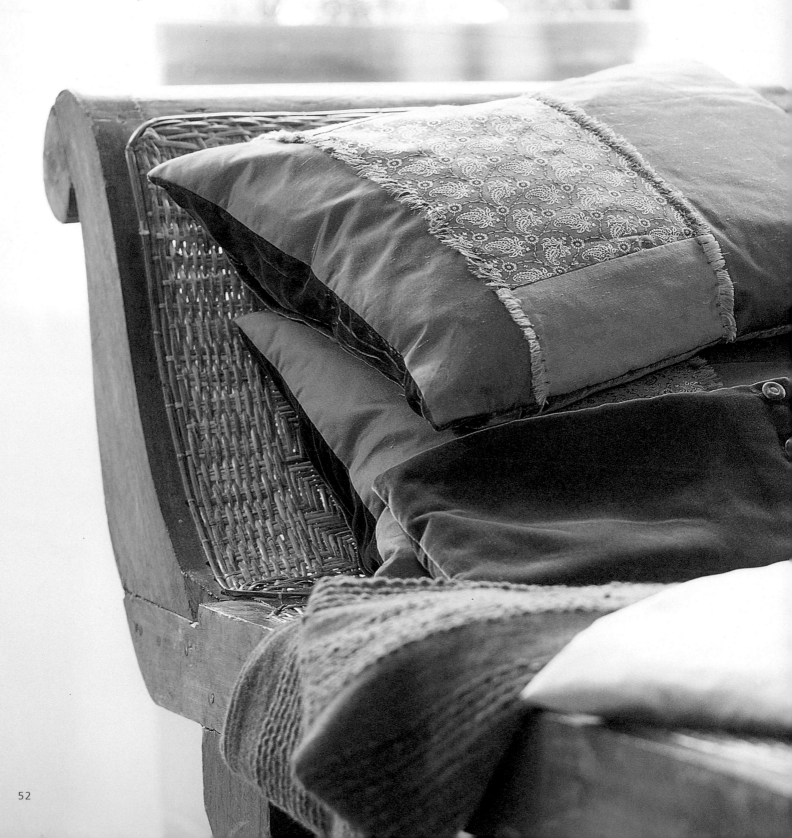

fighting fatigue

Sleep lets us renew and repair ourselves physically, spiritually, and emotionally. Sometimes it evades us when we are most in need of it — we may have overridden our natural tiredness mechanisms and become over-stimulated so that we cannot switch off, or had too many artificial stimulants during the day, such as tea, coffee, and alcohol. Aromatherapy is of use at such times, helping us unwind, while learning to catnap is also a good reenergizing habit to adopt. Short snatches of sleep can provide enough energy to get us through the day and prevent chronic overtiredness from setting in.

Conversely, although rest is a healing necessity at certain times, too much sleep can cause problems. Resultant poor muscle tone, weak circulation, and sluggish metabolism can leave someone lacking in energy and enthusiasm for life. Stimulating and enlivening essences are then of help when bathing or showering, combined with regular massage to stimulate the circulation, improve muscle tone, and lift the spirit, and gentle exercises to reestablish a reasonable level of vitality.

Create an invigorating atmosphere
by using mood-enhancing blends of
essential oils to fill the air around
you with wonderfully energizing
and stimulating fragrances.

refreshing
SURROUNDINGS

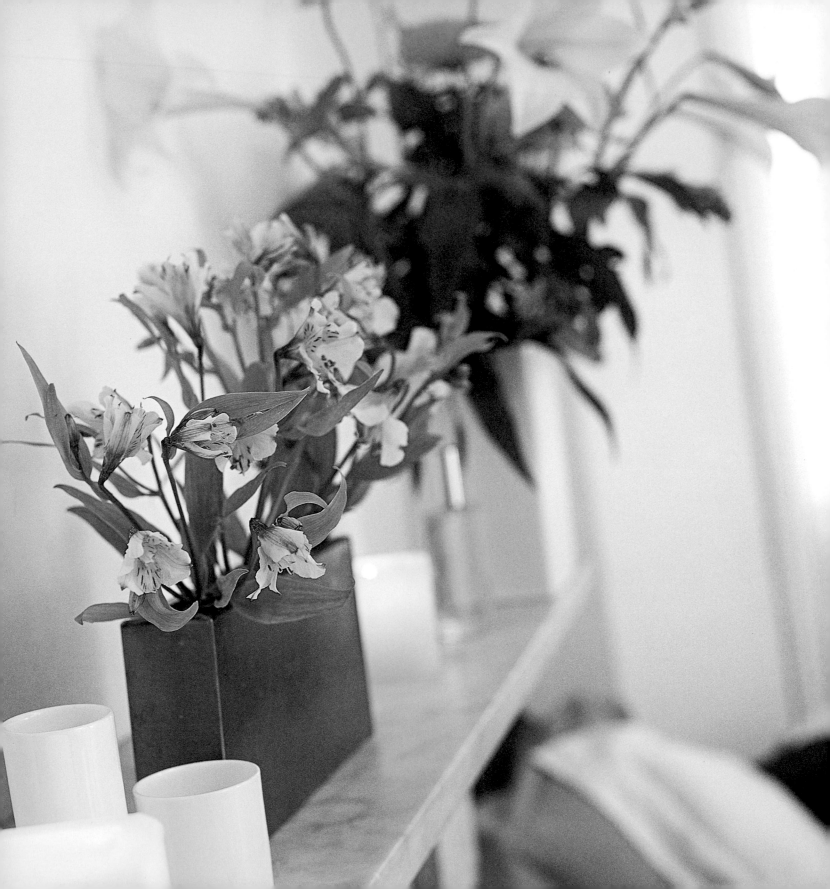

Since our energy levels directly reflect not only our lifestyles

but also where we live, ideally we need an environment that

helps maintain and enhance our levels of vitality. This can

involve aspects of health that are not immediately obvious.

Essentially, we are increasingly assailed by chemicals, which

bombard us on every level. They are used to clean our homes

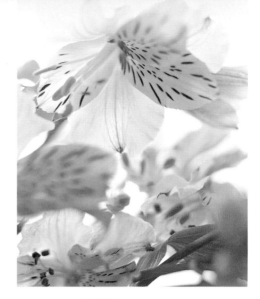

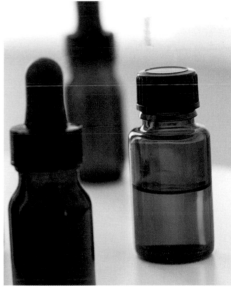

stimulating fragrances for a
reviving atmosphere

and to freshen and scent our environment, to spray on our

bodies and hair, and they occur in our food and drink. The use

of essential oils and holistic principles, therefore, can best help

us revitalize, reenergize, and generally invigorate ourselves and

our environment, at home and at work, using natural methods.

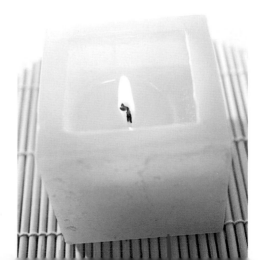

Any room can benefit from the addition of natural aromas, but since the living room is often the most communal room in the house, it is often in need of fragrant refreshing. Whether the atmosphere has been tainted by cigarette smoke or pet smells, or is just generally suffering from family day-to-day living, essential oils can be released into the air to cleanse and scent the atmosphere naturally and effectively.

For immediate effect, use a plant spray filled with water to which you have added a blend of essences (*see* p. 62). Spray it liberally around the room at intervals, especially when dusting or vacuuming. The essences not only impart an energizing aroma, but also have an antiseptic, insect repellent, and mood-enhancing effect – especially relevant for doing housework!

Vaporizers take more time to disperse essential oil fragrances. Traditional models consist of a ceramic bowl, which holds water and a few drops of essence, set over a hollow base housing a small votive candle. As the candle heats the water,

Vaporizers subtly and gently impart the "essential" aroma into the room over a period of time.

the essential oil molecules are vaporized and released into the air. Vaporizers impart the aroma into the room over a period of time measured by the life span of the candle. This method is useful when preparing the room for a particular reason, and the lit candle is attractive but should never be left unattended.

vitalizing vapors

Aromatic atmosphere

Vaporize one of the following blends for an invigorating atmosphere.

Bergamot essence, 6 drops

Cedarwood essence, 3 drops

Rosemary essence, 3 drops

Geranium essence, 4 drops

Rosemary essence, 2 drops

Juniper essence, 2 drops

Housework help

To refresh the air, add one of the following blends to a plant spray containing 4 ounces of water:

Grapefruit essence, 20 drops

Geranium essence, 15 drops

Pine essence, 10 drops

Lime essence, 20 drops

Lemon essence, 20 drops

Juniper essence, 10 drops

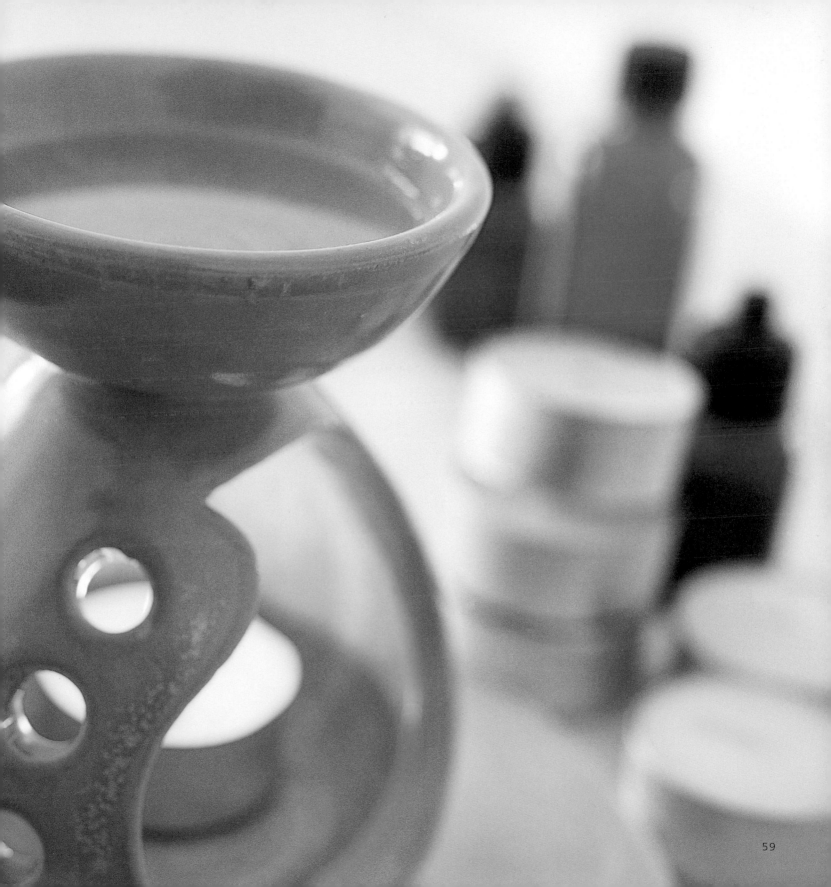

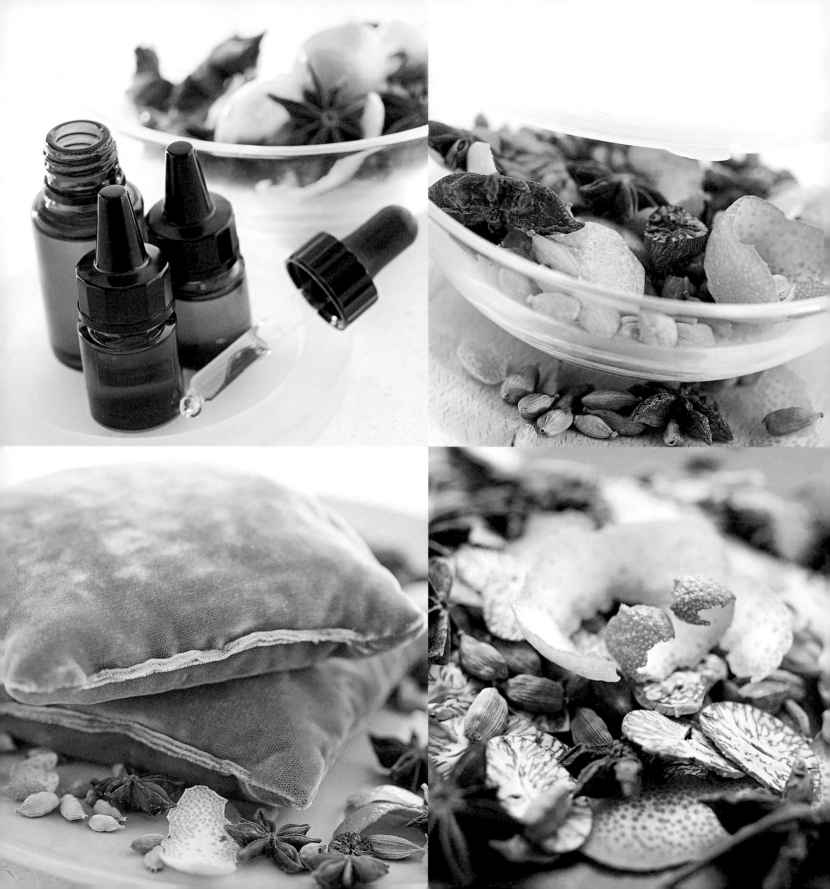

A large bowl of colorful potpourri looks attractive in any room and, with its natural fragrance enhanced by essential oils, helps keep the air fresh by imparting its aroma over a long period of time. The same mixture can also be used to fill small sachets of lightweight fabric to hang on the backs of doors so the revitalizing aroma wafts into the room as the door opens.

Make your own natural potpourri using spices, citrus peel, or aromatic flowers and herbs from the backyard. Dry citrus fruit by placing pieces of peel and slices of fruit on a baking sheet in a very low oven for a few hours until dried out

natural citrus potpourri

Citrus potpourri blend

Mixed dried slices of orange, lemon, and lime, and curled dried peel of 1 lime, 1 lemon, and ½ orange

1 heaped cup geranium leaves

1 heaped cup dried garden flowers

1 heaped cup dried garden herbs

1 tablespoon orris-root powder

Lime essence, 5 drops

Grapefruit essence, 3 drops

Lemon essence, 2 drops

Make the potpourri as for the instructions given in the main text for drying the citrus fruit and plant material and combining all the ingredients.

and hard. They will have no scent, but look attractive in potpourri. Dry herbs and flowers by binding their stems together and hanging them upside down in a warm place. When they are dry, carefully remove the flower heads from the stems. Place all your potpourri ingredients in an airtight container and add 20 drops of your chosen essential oils to every four cups of dried plant matter. Seal the box and leave for at least 48 hours so the mixture becomes impregnated with the aroma of the essences.

Empty the potpourri into a bowl or use it slightly crushed to fill small bags made from squares of cotton, gauze, or other fabric with a wide weave, which allows the essential oil molecules to disperse easily. Secure the sachets with stitching, ribbon, or string. Refresh the potpourri fragrance as necessary by adding drops of oil to the bowl or the sachet fabric.

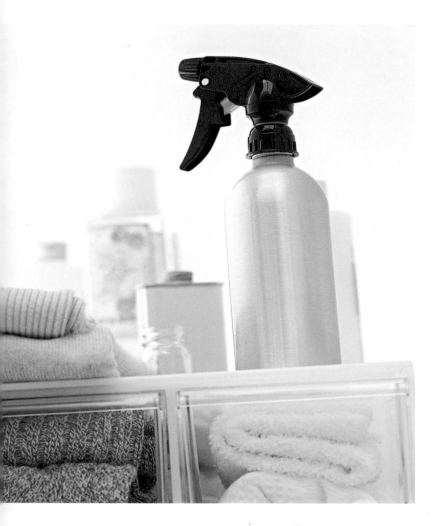

To encourage feelings of vitality in your immediate surroundings, replace any synthetic air freshener — aerosol or otherwise — with a natural one of your own. One easy way is to combine various essential oils and water in a plant spray. Try to find a metal or glass atomizer since these can look attractive and are not adversely affected by essential oils. Remember to shake it well before use to disperse the essences. One of the joys of making your own air freshener is that you can make different combinations for different rooms, according to the ambience you wish to create and the requirements of that room.

In the bedroom a refreshing room spray first thing in the morning can help you waken fully, stimulating your ability to focus on the day ahead. Uplifting essences can also help alleviate that Monday morning feeling, when all you want to do is stay in bed! Since the bedroom is principally the place for rest and recuperation, however, it is advisable to use the stimulant essences only in the morning to make sure they do not adversely affect your sleep pattern.

Essential oils can also be used to scent clothes naturally, and their insect repellent properties help keep moths and other insects at bay. Their delightful fragrance far surpasses any synthetic chemical substitute — especially mothballs! Make three to six sachets (*see* p. 61), depending on the size of your closet, complete with ties from which to hang the sachets on coat hangers or hooks. Fill the sachets with the dried material of your choice — flowers and herbs, whole spices such as cloves and cinnamon sticks, citrus peel, or tiny pine cones, all of which look attractive when seen through the sachet material — and to which you can add your favorite essences.

a zest for living

Morning reviver spray

Spraying uplifting essences can help refresh your surroundings and counteract tiredness and apathy when you first wake up. Add one of the following blends to a plant spray containing 4 ounces of water:

Bergamot essence, 15 drops

Lime essence, 15 drops

Geranium essence, 10 drops

Geranium essence, 40 drops

Rosemary essence, 20 drops

Juniper essence, 20 drops

Scented clothes sachets

Use one of the following blends
for every 4 cups of dried plant
matter used in your sachets:

Lemon essence, 10 drops
Lime essence, 10 drops

Lime essence, 12 drops
Geranium essence, 8 drops

Cedarwood essence, 15 drops
Eucalyptus essence, 5 drops

*Even at work, essences can lift our mood and
help us maintain our perspective when pressures
are on and tempers are frayed.*

enhancing efficiency

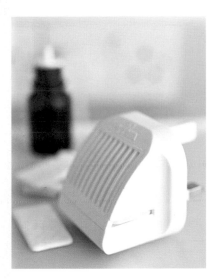

Electric room diffuser

This works by putting a drop or two of essential oil on a tab of thick paper, which is then inserted into a slit in the diffuser. Once it is plugged into an electric socket, the diffuser heats up and releases the essential oil molecules into the room via small vents.

General office invigoration

Add the following to a vaporizer:

Lime essence, 5 drops
Lemon essence, 3 drops
Peppermint essence, 1 drop

Revitalizing essences can be effective in the workplace by helping to enhance surroundings and prevent the spread of infection, a common problem wherever a number of people work in close proximity in an enclosed environment.

Vaporizing certain oils can help maintain concentration and stimulate conversation, energy, and creativity. If the atmosphere is dry, try using humidifiers. Even a simple bowl of water or a small receptacle hung on a radiator provide further opportunities for using essential oils and can help prevent dry, itchy eyes and sore throats.

When you need extra powers of concentration, strong brain stimulants, or cephalics, such as eucalyptus and peppermint, can be effective inhaled directly from the bottle. These are also useful for driving, when concentration is paramount. It is even possible to buy small fans that plug into the cigarette lighter and waft these essential oil molecules at you.

As always, drink plenty of water while at work – you are expending energy so you must rehydrate in order to participate and concentrate effectively. If you crave a hot drink, try mentally stimulating and physically refreshing herb teas, such as fennel or peppermint, with added ginger, honey, or lemon. Other steps to enhance your efficiency include growing large leafy plants, which can impart extra oxygen and take up some of the toxins in your work environment. Also consider using an ionizer to help improve the quality of the air you breathe.

fragrant food

You can grow your own herbs in even the smallest of yards or in windowboxes. Used fresh or dried, herbs add real zest to recipes and can be included in table arrangements to freshen the atmosphere and stimulate conversation.

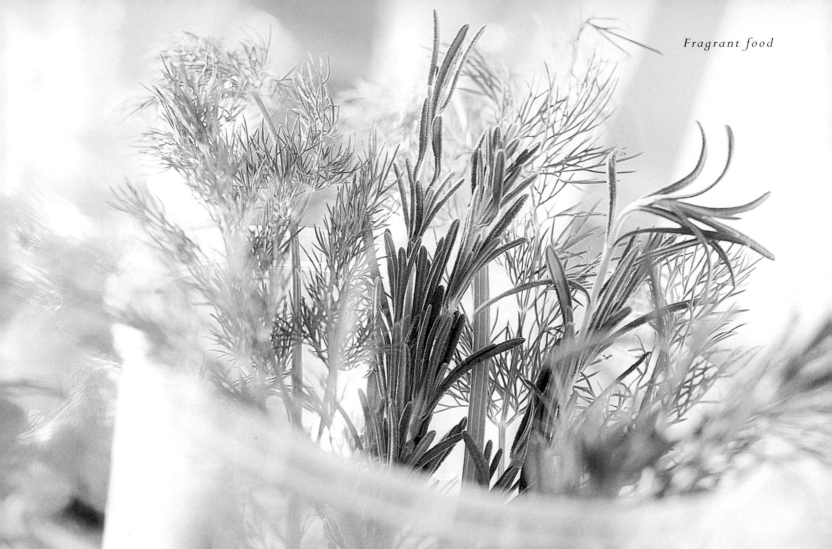

Including herbs in our diet gives us access to the health-giving properties of the essential oils internally without administering them in their concentrated forms. When used in cooking, the herb often has a similar, although not identical, action to the essence used aromatherapeutically. Specific herbs can be used in recipes according to nutritional and medicinal requirements.

Rosemary helps stimulate digestion and circulation. It is particularly useful for its warming, tonic effect in winter and is indicated for tiredness and depression due to overwork. Black pepper has a stimulating effect, useful for fatigue and low immunity, and is a circulatory booster. It is also an expectorant, so it can ease winter coughs and colds, as can ginger, which is a useful digestive aid and can help with travel sickness. Mint has a toning action on the digestion, easing indigestion, trapped gas, hiccups, and sickness. It can also help cold or flu sufferers, easing high temperatures and sore throats, and relieving congestion. Thyme, too, is useful here, being a strong immunity booster, with a particular affinity for the respiratory tract.

sprays & rinses

Kitchen deodorizer

Add to a plant spray

containing 4 ounces of water:

Lime essence, 20 drops

Cedarwood essence, 10 drops

Eucalyptus essence, 5 drops

Kitchen surface cleaner

Add the following to 2 pints of

water and use as a final rinse:

Bergamot essence, 5 drops

Tea tree essence, 3 drops

Eucalyptus essence, 1 drop

Thyme essence, 1 drop

Kitchen floor cleaner

Clean the floor with detergent,

then add the following to 2 pints

of water and use as a final rinse:

Pine essence, 4 drops

Lemon essence, 3 drops

Niaouli essence, 2 drops

Thyme essence, 1 drop

Bathroom bacteria blitzer

Add the following to 4 ounces of

water and use as a spray or soak a

cleaning cloth in the liquid and

squeeze out before using:

Lemon essence, 10 drops

Pine essence, 10 drops

Thyme essence, 5 drops

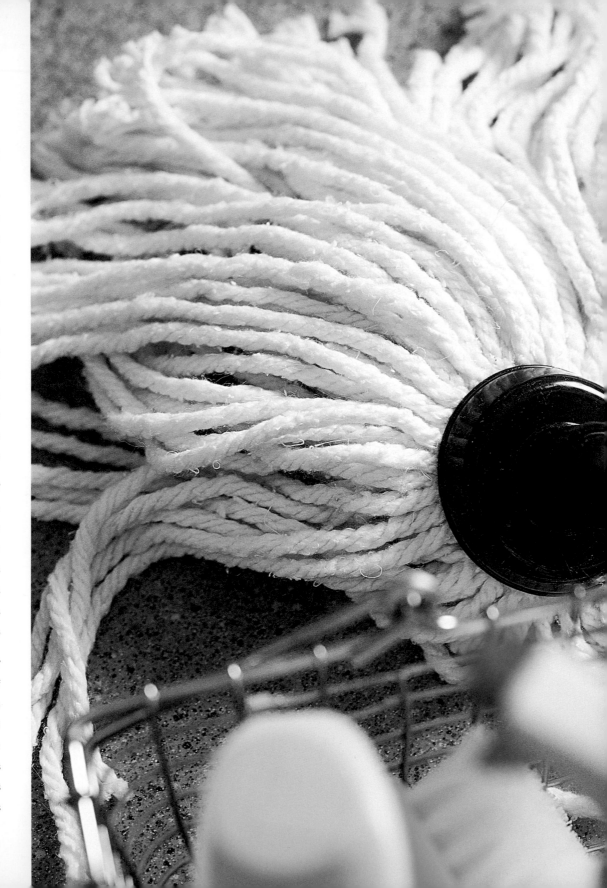

Essential oils are alternatives to commercial cleaning products, and help engender and restore vitality around the home. In the kitchen, they release a tenacious odor against lingering cooking smells and impart antiseptic and antimicrobial properties, qualities equally invaluable for cleaning bathroom surfaces and floors. Add the essences to a plant spray (*see* p. 62) or to a bowl of water in which a cleaning cloth is soaked before use. They help neutralize microbes on external surfaces, as well as those in sinks and drains when the dirty water is poured away. (Essential oils too old for therapeutic use are usable for cleaning since their antiseptic properties can improve with age.)

essential
household cleaning

For other antiseptic and fragrant effects, adding 1 drop of pine essence to the cardboard tube core of a roll of toilet paper effectively scents it. Add 10 drops of lemon or lime essence to 4 ounces of liquid detergent; try cleaning windows in the traditional manner with vinegar and newspaper, then add 1 drop of lemon essence to your final wad of paper or soft cloth to remove streaks. Similarly, after cleaning the fridge, add 2 drops of lemon essence to the final rinse to freshen and deodorize it. Finally, pet bedding requires regular washing. To help reduce animal odors and repel insects, add 2 drops each of juniper, tea tree, and peppermint essence to the final rinse.

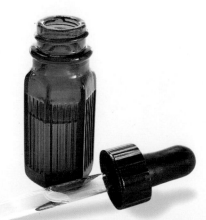

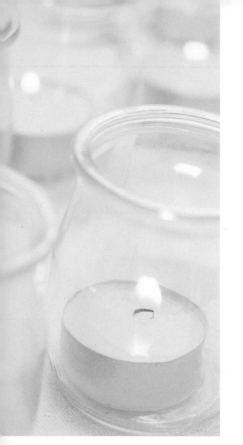

Essential oils can be used to great effect to create a fresh, invigorating atmosphere when you give a party. The room will smell inviting if essences are vaporized or sprayed before guests arrive, and can be used to help stimulate conversation.

For a dinner party, oils such as peppermint and rosemary or lime and juniper, can be vaporized or sprayed after eating rich food, to help cleanse the palette and to clear stale food or smoke odors before the next course is served. If conversation

perfumes for parties

is flagging or tiredness sets in, essential oils such as grapefruit, ginger, and bergamot are effective for accentuating the party atmosphere and maintaining the mood.

To create an aromatic centerpiece for the table, try filling a bowl with pine cones, which have been impregnated with pine and bergamot, cedarwood and lemon, or ginger and lime essence. This can be done by spraying them with a room spray mixture, and leaving the water and oil to sink in and gradually evaporate. If you wish the aroma to be stronger and longer lasting, soak the pine cones in 6 ounces of water to which you have added up to 30 drops of essential oil. Stir regularly to make sure the oils disperse, and soak for 12–24 hours.

At Christmas, these pine cones are ideal suspended on ribbon and hung over mantelpieces, or beams or from curtain rods. Make sure the cones have dried before using them, and take care not to hang them near naked flames.

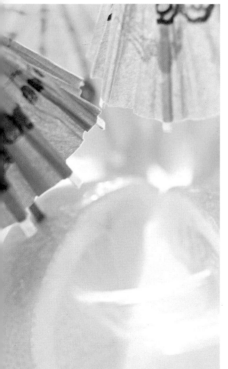

Party room spray

To create a fresh, invigorating
atmosphere and to help stimulate
conversation, add to a plant spray
containing 6 ounces of water:

Geranium essence, 30 drops

Lemon essence, 20 drops

Peppermint essence, 10 drops

A common problem when flying is dehydration, so drink plenty of spring water to help prevent puffy ankles and tiredness. For nausea or tiredness while flying, ginger, peppermint, or grapefruit essence are all helpful inhaled directly from the bottle or as a drop on a tissue. If you are frightened by flying, take Rescue Remedy, one of the Bach flower remedies.

After the flight soak in an aromatic bath to revitalize you. If possible, have a massage to relieve the symptoms of jet lag. The oils to choose will depend on the specific problems, which can include water retention, tiredness, headache, insomnia, swollen ankles, and general lack of "balance."

jet lag travel pack

An invaluable natural energy booster for your travel pack is Siberian ginseng, which comes in the form of capsules containing a standardized dry extract and is widely used as a general tonic. Its restorative, protective, and energizing powers boost the immune system and strengthen stamina and energy levels. It is particularly valuable during periods of intense physical and/or emotional stress and strain, and can be taken safely over a long period of time without negative effects. Make sure you buy the unadulterated version. Commercially grown Chinese and North American ginseng are also available. The former is used as a sexual tonic and the latter for its adaptogenic properties – meaning that it helps the body adapt to certain conditions in order to achieve a state of balance.

after-flight bath & massage oils

For a revitalizing bath, add to 1 teaspoon of vegetable oil:

For the morning: 5 drops of grapefruit, 4 drops of geranium, and 1 drop of eucalyptus essence

For the evening: 5 drops of bergamot, 3 drops of cypress, and 2 drops of juniper essence

For a jet lag-relief massage add to 1 ounce sweet almond oil:

For the morning: 3 drops of rosemary, 2 drops of lemon, and 2 drops of lime essence

For the evening: 5 drops of bergamot, 3 drops of cypress, and 2 drops of geranium essence

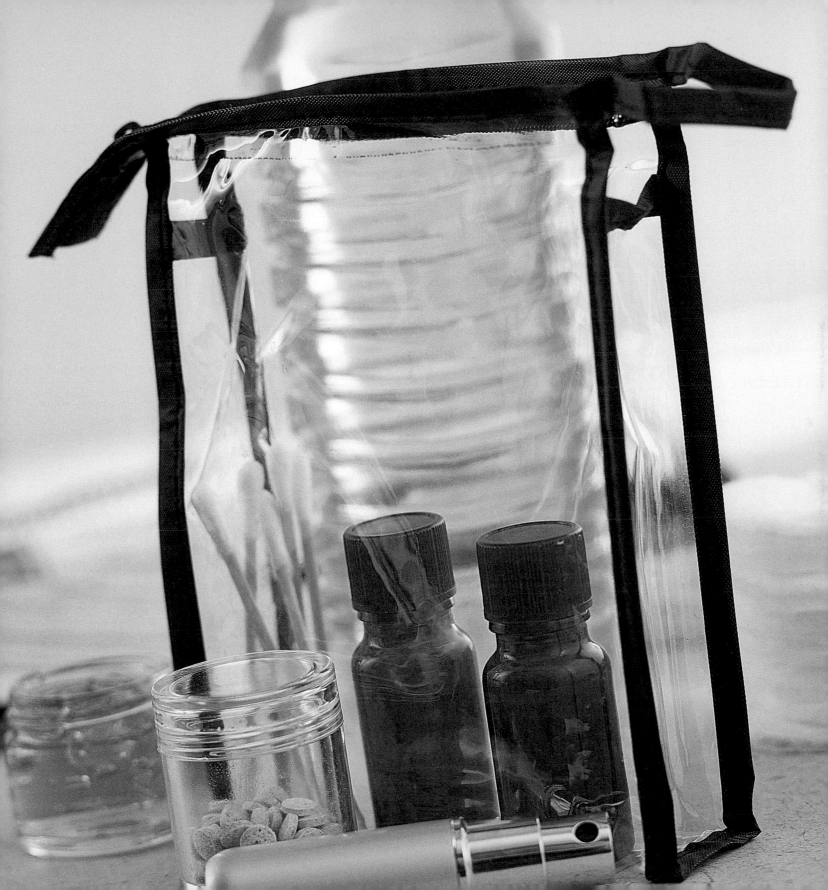

Essential oils are safe, gentle, and profoundly effective, but they are extremely concentrated, and as with any therapeutically powerful substance, they need to be used with respect. Misuse can result in irritation, sensitization, or actual damage to the system – although this is extremely rare. If you adhere to the following guidelines, you will be able to benefit from and enjoy the essential oils to their full potential.

As with many complementary therapies, aromatherapy works effectively alongside orthodox medicine, and in some instances offers a safe and effective form of treatment for many long-term conditions, especially those linked to stress and tension, such as backache, headaches, sleeping problems, and depression, without the side effects of long-term drug use. Orthodox medicine can, however, provide an important life-saving treatment, so a balanced approach between the two is advisable.

- Avoid getting essences in the eye, as this can cause permanent damage. If you do, rinse it with milk and see a doctor immediately. Close eyes during inhalations to avoid irritation.
- Never bring undiluted essential oils into contact with mucus membranes (mouth and respiratory tract and genital-urinary tract), as severe irritation and discomfort may result.
- Certain essential oils should be strictly avoided during pregnancy, including clary sage, black pepper, cedarwood, geranium, marjoram, and jasmine. It is advisable to avoid using any essences in massage during the first three months of pregnancy, and altogether if there is a history of miscarriage. Exceptions are the very gentle rose, neroli, lavender, and camomile, which can all be used safely when diluted: 3–4 drops in baths and 1–2 drops in massage blends. Vaporizing oils is a safe alternative way of using them.

Sensitive skin
- Those with sensitive skin should avoid black pepper, cedarwood, pine, and ginger. Some oils act as sensitizers to hypersensitive skin, so avoid benzoin, jasmine, pine, clary sage, and rose, and ylang ylang at high concentration or very regular application. Sandalwood, jasmine, bergamot, ginger, geranium, lime, and vetiver can cause dermatitis on hypersensitive skin.
- If in doubt, do a skin-patch test first. Prepare the dilution of the oil you wish to test, wash and dry the forearm thoroughly, add a sample of the blend to the gauze of a large bandage, and apply it to the sensitive skin on the inside of the forearm. Leave it for 24 hours unless irritation or discomfort occurs. If the skin is inflamed or irritated after this time, do not use the essence in question. Although this procedure does not guarantee that an adverse reaction will be prevented, it usually indicates

aromatherapy practicalities

General guidelines
- Before using any essential oils, read the contra-indications on pp. 76–8. Some oils are hazardous, so don't use any not covered in this book without professional advice or further reference.
- Each drop of essential oil is highly concentrated, and the majority should be used only when diluted according to the recommendations. Lavender and tea tree are the only oils that can be used undiluted in small amounts.
- Never use more than 10 drops of essence in a bath; clean plastic baths thoroughly after use.
- Do not take oils orally. Serious damage or even death may result if oils are taken internally without professional prescription by an aromatologist or clinical aromatherapist.

- Estrogenic stimulants, such as clary sage and geranium, should be avoided by women suffering from fibroids or uterine, ovarian, or breast cancer.
- Lavender, clary sage, and petitgrain are often recommended for treating asthma, but some asthmatics, especially those with hay fever, may find lavender irritates their condition.
- Keep essential oils out of reach of children. Make sure there is adult supervision at all times; give inhalations for short periods only.
- Always consult a medical practitioner in the event of serious or prolonged illness. This is especially important in the care of babies, children, pregnant women, high temperature, convulsions, concussion, and severe burns.

if an oil is not suited for a particular skin type.
- If you have sensitive skin, dilute essential oils in 1 teaspoon of milk or vegetable oil before adding them to the bath for adequate dilution and dispersal of the oils.
- Babies and the elderly have hypersensitive skin, so concentrated essences should not be used. Dilute 1 drop in a teaspoon of milk for baths and 1 drop (of camomile or lavender) in 1 teaspoon of vegetable oil for massage. Or vaporize the essences or use them in sprays.
- Some oils are phototoxic, making the skin sensitive to ultraviolet light and causing pigmentation. Cedarwood, ginger, and citrus oils like bergamot, mandarin, and orange should be avoided before exposure to sun or a sun bed.

Massage guidelines

- Do not use more than a 2.5 percent dilution unless professionally advised to do so.
- Do not apply deep pressure during massage, especially in the region of the spine, and do not work on any area that is very painful.
- Avoid pressure on the abdomen and lower back during pregnancy. Only use very gentle techniques, especially in the first three months.
- Do not give vigorous whole-body massage on the first two days of menstruation as it can accelerate bleeding; use gentle or localized massage on arms, hands, feet, legs, and face.
- Do not give massage in cases of the following: severe heart disease; very high or low blood pressure; hemorrhaging or a history of blood clotting (stimulating the circulation may cause a blood clot to move); epilepsy (massage with some oils could bring on an attack); high temperature (use cool compresses); serious infection (massage stimulates the circulation, which may cause the infection to spread, and raises the temperature – local application can be used and massage can be beneficial during recuperation, but seek professional advice).
- Avoid the following: site of injury – fractures, open wounds, scar tissue, severe bruising, inflammation, burns or sunburn; infected areas (lavender or tea tree may be effective, but seek professional advice); unidentified lumps (seek medical advice if any are found – they may be fatty tissue, but it is important to check); varicose veins (massage in early stages can help prevent their development).
- Do not massage a subject who has consumed a heavy meal or excessive amounts of alcohol.
- Diabetics can benefit from massage, but only treat those with balanced insulin levels; pay attention to their temperature as they may be insensitive to fluctuations. For those who have been recently diagnosed, seek medical advice.

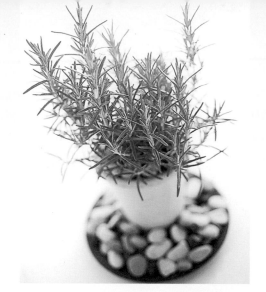

directory of essences

The 18 essential oils featured below are not the only essences that promote a state of vitality, but comprise a comprehensive range of the most profoundly uplifting and revitalizing oils, which can be used to promote and enhance the body's ability to recover and recuperate from modern-day stress. Revitalizing essences can be divided into three main categories, although not all of them fall into these groups:

Antidepressants Bergamot, black pepper, cedarwood, geranium, grapefruit, lime, peppermint and rosemary.

Stimulants Black pepper, cedarwood, cypress, eucalyptus, ginger, lemon, lime, niaouli, peppermint, pine, rosemary and thyme.

Harmonizers Bergamot, geranium and lemon.

Bergamot (*Citrus bergamia*)

This incredibly versatile and universally loved oil is named after the Italian city, Bergamo, where it was originally sold.

Physical properties Its antiseptic, immunity-boosting action is particularly recommended for both genital-urinary and respiratory infections. Its antiviral and antibacterial properties help acne, spots, eczema and psoriasis, cold sores, shingles and chicken pox (in combination with eucalyptus and tea tree). It acts as a digestive stimulant, mild laxative, and analgesic for colitis, trapped gas, and indigestion, and can also be helpful for treating eating disorders and loss of appetite caused by depression.

Emotional properties Helpful for grief, depression, and anxiety. The balancing action promotes calm, controls anger, and increases self-confidence and self-esteem.

Contraindications Phototoxic, so can cause pigmentation on exposure to the sun or a sun bed. Can irritate sensitive skin, especially if the oil is old.

Black pepper (*Piper nigrum*)

The aphrodisiac qualities are due to pepper's warming, stimulating effect, which awakens and enlivens the senses.

Physical properties Its painkilling action relieves muscular aches, neuralgia, toothache, and indigestion. It stimulates the circulation and helps chilblains, bruises, chills, and poor muscle tone. Can also reduce raised temperatures and boost immunity, and has an antiseptic, antimicrobial, expectorant effect that is particularly helpful for chronic catarrhal conditions. Its antispasmodic action stimulates a sluggish digestion and eases constipation, while its diuretic quality helps urinary infections and detoxification. It also stimulates the appetite and boosts energy, and it is indicated for anemia and resultant fatigue.

Emotional properties An antidepressant, it stimulates the emotions and releases suppressed anger and frustration, promoting vitality. Also relieves apathy and indifference.

Contraindications Can irritate sensitive skin, so use in very small amounts (1 drop in baths, 2 drops in massage blends).

Cedarwood (*Juniperus virginiana*)

Probably the first essence ever to be extracted; used extensively by the Egyptians for mummification and in cosmetics and medicines.

Physical properties Its antispasmodic action works on both respiratory and genital-urinary infections. It stimulates the circulation, eases arthritic conditions and lymphatic congestion, has an astringent effect on oily skin and hair, and helps dandruff. In minute doses it can improve eczema, psoriasis, and dermatitis (do a skin-patch test as it can be an irritant). It also soothes insect bites and acts as an insect repellent.

Emotional properties Has an emotionally harmonizing effect, easing tension and aggression, and encouraging relaxation and a meditative outlook.

Contraindications Avoid during pregnancy; may irritate sensitive skin.

Cypress (*Cupressus sempervirens* var. *sticta*)

Cypress was associated with death and the afterlife in ancient Egypt and by the Romans, hence its Latin name *sempervirens*, meaning "ever living."

Physical properties It is an astringent for many form of excess fluids within the body and for skin conditions. Its antispasmodic nature is particularly indicated for asthma, sinusitis, bronchitis, laryngitis, and tickly coughs, for which its antiseptic and decongestant properties also help. It can help relieve muscular cramps and discomfort relating to arthritic and rheumatic conditions, stomach upsets, and period pain. Useful as a hormonal regulator, especially for menstrual problems. Its deodorizing effect helps reduce excessive perspiration; and as a circulatory stimulant, it helps varicose veins, poor circulation, and hemorrhoids.

Emotional properties Spiritually cleansing, purifying, and protecting. Has a calming effect on uncontrollable tears and hysteria. Indicated for stress-related conditions and nervousness resulting in bouts of anger and frustration.

Contraindications Avoid during pregnancy. Avoid if suffering from high blood pressure or cancer.

Eucalyptus (*Eucalyptus globulus*)

The Aborigines were the first to use the antiseptic qualities of eucalyptus and bound wounds with fresh leaves.

Physical properties A strong stimulant, it helps clear mental fatigue and headaches and assist concentration. Its antimicrobial properties make it effective in assisting recovery from colds, coughs, flu, chicken pox, high temperature, and even malaria and typhoid. It is strongly recommended in preventive measures when illness is in the locality. Its decongestant/expectorant properties assist catarrhal congestion. An antifungal agent and a diuretic, eucalyptus is also indicated for urinary infections. It has use as a local painkiller in combination with bergamot, and is also useful for burns, blisters, and skin infections. Muscular aches and pains and arthritic conditions can benefit from massage with diluted eucalyptus. It is a strong insect repellent.

Emotional properties It can be used to purify or cleanse a negative atmosphere or an area tainted by anger or conflict.

Contraindications Avoid if suffering from high blood pressure or epilepsy, or if undergoing homeopathic treatment. Not for use by babies or young children; store it out of their reach as small internal doses can be fatal. Only ever use tiny amounts (1 drop per ounce massage oil base, 1 drop per inhalation or bath)

Fennel (*Foeniculum vulgare*)

Fennel was used extensively in the past for animal fodder, to ward off evil spirits, and to improve eyesight.

Physical properties Aids digestion and calms nausea, gas, hiccups, indigestion. Helps relieve constipation. Its diuretic properties ease premenstrual water retention and urinary infections. It is indicated for the treatment of cellulite, and its detoxifying effects are useful after too much alcohol and cigarettes. Its hormonally regulating effect helps regulate scanty menstruation, ease period pain and premenstrual syndrome. For nursing mothers, fennel can help increase the flow of milk.

Emotional properties Emotionally revitalizing and strengthening; spiritually protecting. Eases nervous tension and stress-related asthma or wheezing.

Contraindications Avoid during pregnancy and if suffering from epilepsy. Not for use by children under the age of six. Use sweet rather than bitter fennel to avoid skin sensitization.

Geranium (*Pelargonium graveolens*)

Has many physical and emotional uses.

Physical properties Balances various functions of the body, for example has an astringent effect on oily skin but promotes renewal and repair of dry and mature skin and some forms of dermatitis, eczema, and shingles. Stimulates the circulation and has a diuretic action, which helps relieve fluid retention, lymphatic sluggishness, cellulitis, urinary infections, and gallstones. Can help premenstrual syndrome, tender breasts, and hot flashes.

Emotional properties Balances emotional extremes linked to the menstrual cycle or stress. Lifts the mood and refreshes the spirits.

Contraindications Avoid during the first three months of pregnancy.

Ginger (*Zingiber officinale*)

Used by many ancient civilizations to improve sexual prowess.

Physical properties Its painkilling, antispasmodic, antiseptic action relieves respiratory infections, indigestion, constipation, arthritic, rheumatic and muscular aches, stomach ache, backache, toothache, and varicose veins. Helps relieve nausea, hangovers, and tiredness, and stimulates appetite. Regulates menstrual cycle; aids impotence and frigidity.

Emotional properties The warming aphrodisiac effect promotes sensuality and relieves nervous exhaustion and apathy.

Contraindications Use in very small quantities, as the scent can overpower other essences; may irritate sensitive skin.

Grapefruit (*Citrus paradisi*)

Can be helpful in the treatment of eating disorders such as anorexia and bulimia.

Physical properties Its detoxifying, properties stimulate the liver and gall bladder, aid digestion, and enhance lymphatic circulation. Mildly diuretic, it

increases urine flow and helps relieve water retention, cellulite, and excess weight related to congestion of the system by assisting with the breakdown of fats. Can help reduce high blood pressure and may be useful for stress-induced headaches, migraine, PMS, and for alcohol or drug withdrawal.

Emotional properties Helpful for depression related to frustration and irritability, especially for those who eat for comfort. Emotionally cleansing, refreshing, and revitalizing. Helps alleviate doubt and self-reproach, releasing disappointment, and disillusionment, and promoting self-belief and confidence.

Contraindications Unlike other citrus essences, grapefruit is not phototoxic, but it can become irritant and sensitizing if oxidized. Use within six months of purchase, thereafter for vaporizing only.

Juniper (berry) (*Juniperus communis*)

A highly versatile essence, it was used by ancient civilizations to ward off evil.

Physical properties Good for detoxifying. Particularly beneficial for cellulite, fluid retention, varicose veins, arthritis, and gout. It stimulates the release of digestive juices and helps relieve indigestion, trapped gas, and mild stomach upsets; helps recovery from overindulgence. Its astringent and antiseptic nature is useful for treating greasy hair, oily skin and some forms of eczema, dermatitis, psoriasis, and acne.

Emotional properties Energetic cleanser, physically and emotionally. Can be used to purify an area before meditation or relaxation, or to rid an atmosphere of negativity. A general tonic for nervous tension, anxiety, poor memory, jet lag, or general lack of mental clarity.

Contraindications Avoid during pregnancy; not for use by babies or young children, or anyone with kidney

disease or acute kidney or bladder infections. Use with care on sensitive skin. Do not use constantly for prolonged periods.

Lemon (*Citrus limonum*)

Traditionally used to scent clothes and repel insects.

Physical properties Very strong antibacterial, antiseptic agent. Useful sickroom vaporizer for helping stop spread of infection. Its immunity-boosting action helps speed up recovery from illness, as lemon stimulates white blood cell production – the body's defense mechanisms. Its decongestant action is indicated for bronchitis, flu, coughs, and colds. Has a detoxifying, neutralizing effect on excessive acidity in the joints (arthritis, gout, rheumatism) and in the digestive tract (dyspepsia, ulcers). Aids digestion; stimulates and tones pancreas, stomach, liver, and gall bladder; and its diuretic nature helps deal with water retention, especially relating to poor circulation. Its astringent, toning effect is useful for varicose veins, hemorrhoids, broken veins, and cellulite. It can help high blood pressure; helps counteract anemia; and its astringent nature helps rebalance an excessive sebum output leading to oily skin and spots.

Emotional properties Helps promote clarity of thought and vision and a subtle, spiritual awareness; and eases mental argument, conflict, or confusion.

Contraindications Can irritate sensitive skin and is phototoxic, so do not use before exposure to the sun or a sun bed. Older, more oxidized oils have increased potential for sensitization. Use oil within six months for diluted normal application, thereafter use only for vaporizing.

Lime (*Citrus aurantiifolia*)

Refreshing and revitalizing, lime can be helpful in the treatment of alcoholism and anorexia nervosa.

Physical properties Its antiseptic properties work well on respiratory infections, coughs, colds, and flu; it also reduces fever. Its antispasmodic action is helpful for muscle weakness, spasms, and inflammation caused by strain or tension. It can ease stomach cramps caused by anxiety or upset; also helps cellulite, poor circulation, and detoxification.

Emotional properties An uplifting and refreshing antidepressant, which helps to counteract anxiety, fatigue, and listlessness and to restore a sense of perspective.

Contraindications Can irritate sensitive skin and is phototoxic, so do not use before exposure to the sun or a sun bed.

Niaouli (*Melaleuca viridiflora*)

Its antiseptic properties make it a good sick-room spray when diluted in water.

Physical properties Helps any condition with chronic catarrhal congestion, while its anti-inflammatory, analgesic effects help ease the discomfort. As a painkiller, it helps ease joint inflammation, arthritis, and rheumatism. Its antiseptic immuno-stimulant action also indicated for urinary infections. As a digestive and liver tonic, it helps relieve discomfort from trapped gas, diarrhea, gastric and duodenal ulcers. Indicated for asthma, especially when triggered by an allergic response. Can help relieve oily skin, acne, insect bites, and fungal infections (athlete's foot).

Emotional properties Helps revive and refresh spirit and emotions – aids concentration and clear thinking. Indicated for nervous depression.

Contraindications Avoid during pregnancy. Not for use by babies or young children, nor on sensitive skin.

Peppermint (*Mentha piperita*)

A strong brain stimulant, peppermint should only be used in the evenings if you wish to stay alert all night.

Physical properties A renowned digestive aid, it helps relieve pain and inflammation in the stomach and intestines (indigestion, colic, diarrhea, irritable bowel, nausea, vomiting, stomach ache). It is also a liver tonic and has a cooling, anti-inflammatory effect on high temperature when used as a cold compress. Its analgesic effect is also helpful for muscular strain and pain, toothache, and especially neuralgia. A strong brain stimulant, it can be helpful for treating shock or fainting, as well as for reviving mental capacities when fatigue or apathy set in. Inhalation can help relieve motion sickness and vertigo.

Emotional properties Helps invigorate mind and spirit and boosts energy levels.

Contraindications Avoid during pregnancy and lactation; keep away from babies and young children as can cause spasm/choking. Can irritate sensitive skins. Only use very diluted (1 drop per teaspoon bath oil blend, 1 drop per ounce massage oil base); do not use undiluted.

Pine (*Pinus sylvestris*)

The essence is more likely to irritate the skin due to oxidation as it ages.

Physical properties A powerful antiseptic, decongestant, and expectorant, particularly good for the respiratory system (colds, coughs, flu, bronchitis, sinusitis, even pneumonia) when used in inhalations. A circulatory stimulant, it eases joint and muscle pain, arthritic and rheumatic conditions, sciatica, gout (with juniper), and water retention. It also helps symptoms of ME and reduces excessive sweating of the feet, while the diuretic action aids urinary infections. Acts as a tonic and stimulant for prostate problems and impotency.

Emotional properties Its uplifting and refreshing effect helps relieve symptoms of stress and nervous exhaustion. Boosts low self-esteem and self-confidence.

Contraindications Avoid use in massage or baths if suffering from sensitive skin or prostate cancer.

Rosemary (*Rosmarinus officinalis*)

A strong mental stimulant, it is not recommended for use before bedtime.

Physical properties Useful for acute concentration, especially studying, and for mental exhaustion. A circulatory tonic, it stimulates the blood flow, easing tension, stiffness, cramps, and muscular pain, and is useful before and after exercise for stretching muscles. The analgesic effect combined with increase in blood flow (and antispasmodic action) is useful in treating rheumatism, arthritis, painful periods, and headaches. It is also indicated for water retention and varicose veins. For respiratory ailments (sinusitis, tonsillitis, asthma, colds, flu), it is a powerful antimicrobial agent and can be used to relieve congestion and clear the head. A digestive aid, it helps relieve gas, sluggish digestion, and diarrhea. Can stimulate poor liver function and normalize high cholesterol levels. For poor hair condition, stress-related premature hair loss, and dandruff, rosemary can help improve hair condition. Its astringent nature also helps improve greasy hair. In addition, it is indicated for increasing/normalizing low blood pressure and for temporary loss of nerve function or numbness.

Emotional properties Indicated especially for depression linked to fatigue and exhaustion, for apathy and sluggishness, and for periods of convalescence following ill health.

Contraindications Avoid during pregnancy; avoid if suffering from epilepsy or high blood pressure, or if undergoing homeopathic treatment. May irritate sensitive skins. Do not use more than 2–3 drops per ounce massage oil base.

Tea tree (*Melaleuca alternifolia*)

A uniquely versatile medicinal oil.

Physical properties Effective against virus, bacteria, and fungi, it is useful for a variety of ailments – colds, flu, bronchitis, sinusitis, tonsillitis, whooping cough, dandruff, athlete's foot, acne, warts, ringworm, chicken pox, shingles, and urinary infections. Can be applied undiluted in tiny amounts with caution to spots, stings, cuts, plantar warts, and cold sores, etc. – do a skin-patch test if in doubt. An immune stimulant, it helps prevent infection when resistance is low, especially candida (thrush, stomach upsets, etc.), and for speeding up the healing process.

Emotional properties A useful stimulant for shock, nervous exhaustion, and hysteria; a morale booster.

Contraindications Can irritate skin when used above one percent dilution on sensitive skin types. Many adverse reactions are caused by adulterated versions of the genuine essence.

Thyme (*Thymus vulgaris*)

There are over 300 different varieties of thyme. For a kinder, less harsh thyme, *Thymus vulgaris* C T linalol can be used.

Physical properties Its strongly antimicrobial, expectorant nature indicates use for bronchitis, pneumonia, colds, coughs, and flu (inhaled with eucalyptus and others). Its circulatory stimulatory effect is useful for arthritis, rheumatism, sciatica, muscular aches and pains. Helps to raise low blood pressure and to fight infection by stimulating white blood cell production. Useful for treating lethargy and apathy, and during convalescence.

Emotional properties Strengthens and restores vitality and general sense of self.

Contraindications Avoid during pregnancy; avoid if suffering from high blood pressure or sensitive skin. Always dilute before use and use only in minute doses (1 drop per ounce massage oil base).

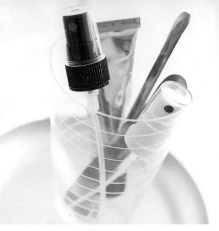

acknowledgments

I would like to thank, as always, my family and friends, who have supported and encouraged me consistently through what have been particularly challenging times! Dominique and James Colthurst, Barbara Day, Miranda Dowie, Lisa Rutter, Emily Bone, Sheila Coote, Philip Tanswell, Sharon Sheargold, Diana Thomas, Emma Corke and Jean Rodgers have all brought their own particular gifts to me exactly when they were most needed, and I will always count myself lucky to know them.

Karen Sheargold deserves a gold medal for the midnight oil she has burnt, and has been great to work with. Charles Wells from Essentially Oils has been a mine of sometimes obscure information, which he consistently relays with kindness and good humour.

I would also like to thank Jean Marshall, who first introduced me to the wonderful world of natural medicine, and consequently saved and redirected my entire life to date. Maria Ball at the Raworth Centre, Dorking, will always receive my thanks and appreciation for the excellent foundation my original aromatherapy training represented 10 years ago and for her continued advice, support and encouragement.

Publisher's Acknowledgments

The publishers would like to thank Frazer Cunningham and Kimberley Watson for allowing us to photograph in their homes, and Sue Parker for producing pages 20 to 23.

index